T0222236

Perinatal Mental Health

a sourcebook for health professionals

Diana Riley
Consultant Obstetric Liaison Psychiatrist,
Aylesbury Vale Community Healthcare NHS Trust and
The South Buckinghamshire NHS Trust

With a Foreword by

Channi Kumar
Professor of Perinatal Psychiatry, Bethlem Royal and
Maudsley Hospitals

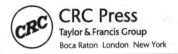

CRC Press
Taylor & Francis Group
Boca Raton London New York

CRC Press is an imprint of the
Taylor & Francis Group, an **informa** business

First published 1995 by Radcliffe Publishing

Published 2016 by CRC Press
Taylor & Francis Group
6000 Broken Sound Parkway NW, Suite 300
Boca Raton, FL 33487-2742

© 1995 by Taylor & Francis Group, LLC
CRC Press is an imprint of Taylor & Francis Group, an Informa business

No claim to original U.S. Government works

ISBN-13: 978-1-87090-578-7 (pbk)

Visit the Taylor & Francis Web site at
http://www.taylorandfrancis.com

and the CRC Press Web site at
http://www.crcpress.com

British Library Cataloguing in Publication Data

A catalogue record for this book is available from the British Library.

Library of Congress Cataloging-in-Publication Data is available.

Typeset by Acorn Bookwork, Salisbury, Wiltshire

Contents

Foreword

There are signs of an awakening interest in the psychiatric problems that occur in childbearing women. Nevertheless, despite knowledge of the sometimes devastating effects on maternal health and adjustment of conditions such as postnatal depression and postpartum psychosis, and an awareness of repercussions in the developing child, the resources allocated to preventing and alleviating such problems are pitiful. In a recent government report on the encouragement of choice and the recognition of the mother as an individual within the context of midwifery care (*Cumberlege Report*. HMSO, London, 1993), the subject of postnatal illness merits ten lines in 108 pages.

Fortunately, much is being done to educate professionals as well as consumers, and this book by Dr Diana Riley should immediately find its way on to the bookshelves of general practitioners, health visitors, midwives, social workers, psychiatrists and – dare one say it – obstetricians. It is the balanced distillation of many years' experience of a dedicated clinical psychiatrist who has provided a model comprehensive service for pregnant and parturient women. Her knowledge comes through in the writing, which is always informative and clear and jargon free. It is also up to date and it will provide an easy but thorough introduction for any professional wishing to know more about psychiatric problems and motherhood; and most important of all, the reader will find sensible advice in every section on how to set about dealing with such problems.

I am often asked to recommend review articles or books to people who are starting in this field as therapists or as researchers, and sometimes for mothers who want to know more. Dr Riley has solved my problem.

Professor Channi Kumar
October 1994

Introduction

Even allowing for the present trend towards smaller families, pregnancy is a common event. Pregnant and postnatal women will make up a substantial part of the work-load of all general practitioners. For example, a practice of 2 000 patients will include about 25 pregnancies each year, and a health district with a population of 500 000 will have over 5 000 deliveries per year. Peripartum care is therefore part of everyday work for general practitioners, midwives and obstetricians. It is not so for mothers, who will experience it only perhaps once or twice in a lifetime, and for whom it will be a memorable and momentous occasion.

As a result of better obstetric care, childbirth has become physically safer over recent years, with maternal and child mortality falling to an all time low. Women are also now largely in control of their own fertility, limiting the number of pregnancies in a way not available to previous generations. They are also perhaps better educated and more articulate about their expectations of pregnancy and delivery, so that each birth experience carries an even greater emotional loading.

However, the emphasis of most antenatal and postnatal care has not kept pace with these developments, and still seems to concentrate exclusively on the physical health of the mother and child, whilst the emotional impact of such an important life event receives little attention.

This book is an attempt to raise awareness in those working in both primary care and obstetric hospital settings of the frequency and importance of the emotional aspects of pregnancy and childbirth. Until this becomes an integral part of professional care for all women, the physically healthy mother and child may well continue to suffer from emotional disorders which, even if mild in nature, may be prolonged and damaging to the individual, to the relationship with a partner, and to the psychological, and even the physical development of the child.

Traditionally, the more serious of these postnatal disorders have been treated by psychiatrists, whilst many of the milder illnesses have gone unrecognized or inadequately treated in the community. There is now increasing evidence that vulnerable women can be identified in the antenatal clinic, and that intervention by the primary care team before delivery can prevent, or at least lessen, the severity of postnatal psychiatric problems. Adequate treatment and support postpartum can also reduce long-term morbidity for both mother and child.

These pregnancy related illnesses form a significant proportion of all psychiatric morbidity seen in general and psychiatric practice. The figures speak for themselves.

- Between 15% and 20% of all patients seen by maternity services have problems related to their mental health which may need to be taken into account in their obstetric management[1].

- More than 10% of all pregnant women score highly enough on screening questionnaires to be considered 'cases' of depression[2,3], although few will be identified as such.

- Between 10% and 20% of newly delivered women will become clinically depressed in the subsequent year; 2% will be referred to a psychiatrist[1].

- Two per thousand recently delivered mothers will need admission to a psychiatric unit.

- Ten per cent of all new female patients referred to psychiatric services have a baby under one year of age, and 25% a child under the age of five.

- Women have 16 times the normal risk of psychiatric admission in the first 30 days postpartum. For women having a first baby by caesarian section, the risk of admission to hospital with a psychotic illness within the first postpartum month is 35 times higher than at other times[4].

Although these very high risks are relatively short-lived, the relative risk for depressive illness in mothers is increased for up to two years postpartum[4].

These important issues can be dealt with by workers in primary care, and most women would certainly prefer an approach from professionals they already know, rather than being referred to a psychiatrist with all the social stigma that this entails. Indeed, there is no other time in a woman's life when she is under such close scrutiny from her general practitioner, midwife and health visitor, or a time when there are so many golden opportunities for helpful intervention.

A psychotherapist[5] wrote in 1989:

> 'A comprehensive mental health service must be based above all on prevention. It must also provide treatment for those who have escaped the preventative net. Prevention must depend first and foremost on the availability of appropriate help to those who care for children – especially mothers of babies.'

He goes on to state that health visitors are ideally placed to be the 'front-line troops', and that, in the course of their ordinary duties, they could enable mothers to get things right from the start, thus avoiding problems for which they might otherwise need (but probably fail to receive) more specialized treatment.

It therefore makes both humanitarian and economic sense to recognize, at an early stage of pregnancy, those who are particularly vulnerable, use preventative measures whenever possible, and identify and treat energetically and immediately, those who slip through the preventative net. This book is an attempt to give all those involved the skills necessary to do this.

References

1. Report of the General Psychiatry Section Working Party on Postnatal Mental Illness. (1992) *Psychiatric Bulletin.* **16**: 519–22.

2. Kumar R and Robson KM. (1984) A prospective study of emotional disorders in childbearing women. *British Journal of Psychiatry.* **144**: 35–47.

3. Hrasky M and Morice R. (1986) The identification of psychiatric disturbance in an obstetric and gynaecological population. *Australian and New Zealand Journal of Psychiatry.* **20**: 63–9.

4. Kendell R, Chalmers JC and Platz C. (1987) Epidemiology of puerperal psychoses. *British Journal of Psychiatry.* **150**: 662–73.

5. Woodmansey AC. (1989) Reversing the vicious spiral: a radical approach to mental health. *British Journal of Clinical and Social Psychiatry.* **6**: 103–6.

1   Pregnancy

There is a popular image of the pregnant woman as 'blooming', with improved physical and emotional health. This is often far from the truth. A particularly notable finding is that women vary enormously in their response to pregnancy, and there is a similar variation with each stage of pregnancy, so that professionals need to be sensitive to women's differing needs for emotional support at any particular time.

There is evidence that some pregnancies may be related to neurotic symptoms. A study of students found that those who became pregnant had a higher incidence of previous consultations for psychiatric problems[1]. Pregnancy may be entered into as an attempt to gain attention, as an escape from an unwelcome situation, to mend a failing relationship, or to provide a love object. Worst of all, and most likely to fail, is the expectation that the child will provide the love and care that the woman has lacked in her life so far.

Joan Raphael-Leff[2] has identified three groups of 'problem pregnancies'. These are:

- conflicted, where the pregnancy is unplanned, untimely, or wrong. This can be as a result of a transient or unhappy relationship, sometimes even as a result of rape or incest. The timing can be wrong, as in the woman who is resentful about the interruption of her career, or a pregnancy too soon after a stillbirth or neonatal death, whilst she is still grieving. A frequent pattern is a pregnancy soon after a termination or miscarriage in an attempt to 'replace' the lost child.

- complicated, by physical or socio-economic problems, or adverse life events. Pregnancies complicated by antepartum haemorrhage or pregnancy induced hypertension, which require the mother to rest in bed for long periods can be tedious and worrying. Where there are serious practical problems with housing, finance, or lack of support from friends or family, the mother will feel insecure and anxious. The 'new house, new baby' is a case in point. Bereavement, perhaps the loss of a parent, during the pregnancy will complicate the mother's feelings, and often leads to postponement of the grieving process until after the birth.

• emotionally sensitized, in which the pregnancy is over- or undervalued because of the previous experience of the woman or her close family members, or due to her own neurotic traits. A previous history of infertility, for example, may mean that the mother overvalues the pregnancy, having unreal expectations about how wonderful it will be, yet being unprepared for the responsibility of a child. Previous pregnancy loss may lead to her withholding attachment to the baby until after the birth.

Psychiatric Problems in Pregnancy

There is a surprising incidence of measurable psychiatric morbidity, even during an apparently 'normal' pregnancy. A prospective study in a London antenatal clinic using the General Health Questionnaire (GHQ) showed that 16% of women were 'cases' of depression at 12–14 weeks into the pregnancy, and that this severity of depression correlated with previous psychological problems, ambivalence about the pregnancy, previous termination and marital tension[3]. A similar Australian survey found an even higher incidence (40%) at 33–34 weeks[4]. Another survey of 179 women at a booking clinic showed that 35% were high scorers on the GHQ, and 29% were confirmed as 'cases' at interview[5]. This is no artefact of questionnaire response. When the women studied are those with 'high risk' pregnancies in terms of physical complications, 66% are found to have a clear psychiatric diagnosis[6].

This degree of morbidity in pregnant women does not seem to be given sufficient recognition by professional carers, perhaps because the emotional condition is thought to be as self-limiting as the physical state, but more likely, because it is not identified or is attributed to a 'normal' overemotional state in pregnancy (*see* Case Study 1.1).

It may, however, have relevance to the outcome of pregnancy. For example, late booking or poor attendance at the antenatal clinic is one way in which the mother's emotional state may influence fetal health. There is also some evidence that physical complications are more frequent in emotionally disturbed women. One study[7] has shown anxiety in pregnancy to correlate with pregnancy induced hypertension, and another[8] that anxious women are more likely to opt for elective induction of labour. Research also shows that women with significant adverse life events (and hence increased stress) in the year preceding delivery are more likely to suffer premature labour[9].

A special case is that of pregnant women who have suffered from previous psychotic illness. Careful follow-up studies show that in general they also vary in their reactions to pregnancy. About 30% report some improvement in their mental health, most of these being in the older age group, and with previous depressive or manic-depressive illness. Negative effects were associated with lack of social support, situational problems and interpersonal difficulties[10]. Psychotic episodes can, and do, occur during pregnancy but are relatively rare compared with their serious increase in frequency and severity postpartum.

Previous neurotic illness has been examined less closely, but there is some evidence to show that panic disorder and obsessive-compulsive symptoms actually improve during pregnancy, only to worsen again after delivery. Women with previous anorexia often react badly to the changing body shape associated with pregnancy, and will be preoccupied with weight and diet.

On the positive side, the incidence of suicide in pregnancy is extremely low. Over a 12-year period, 14 suicides were reported, mostly in the second trimester, whereas the expected number was 281; thus, pregnant women have only 5% of the expected risk of suicide. The numbers were highest in the 15–29 age groups[11].

Society seems to assume that all women will feel equally happy and fulfilled as soon as the pregnancy is established, but even the most stable and mature mother will have times of self-doubt and trepidation, and will need support for herself in order to deal with the demands of her new and unfamiliar role. Some of the 'normal' positive and negative responses are summarized

First trimester
  Pleasure at fulfilment or reproductive role
  Increased status and attention from family and friends
  Successful transition to adulthood
  Increased feeling of well-being
  Sharing an experience with her own mother
Second trimester
  Increasing attachment to the fetus
  Pleasure at quickening and seeing baby on scan
  Increasing detachment from work commitments
  Social acceptance by other mothers
  Beginning preparations for the birth
Third trimester
  Realistic anxiety and pleasure at impending delivery
  Making stronger links with other mothers
  Increasing attachment to her own mother
  Coming to terms with loss of status and income from work
  'Nesting' activities

Table 1.1 Positive changes in pregnancy

in Tables 1.1, 1.2. Most women will fluctuate between these positive and negative feelings at different stages of the pregnancy depending on their own personality, past experience, and socio-cultural setting.

Contributory Factors to Psychological Problems in Pregnancy

A woman's reaction to the confirmation of pregnancy varies with her socio-cultural milieu. For example, the status of pregnancy in society is different in some ethnic and religious groups, and will also vary with time, the size of the existing family, and perhaps even the sex of the existing children.

Support from the partner has been shown in many studies to be an important factor in emotional health during pregnancy. Those experiencing depression commonly report relationship problems, and there is clearly a need in pregnancy, above all

First trimester
  Rejection of, or ambivalence to, pregnancy
  Perception of fetus as 'invasive' and unwelcome
  Adoption of 'invalid' status
  Fear of fetal abnormality; guilt about alcohol, smoking
  Anxiety about repeat of miscarriage, perinatal death
  Guilt about previous termination
  Competitiveness with own mother
Second trimester
  Dislike of changing shape, especially if previously anorexic or
    bulimic
  Public awareness of sexual activity
  Perceived loss of attractiveness; low self-esteem, possible morbid
    jealousy syndrome
  Withdrawal of attachment to fetus if threatened by pregnancy com-
    plications
  Resentment at limitation of activity and leaving work
  Loneliness in home situation; envy of partner's and peer group's
    continuing work role
Third trimester
  Phobic anxiety about labour, pain or hospitals
  Fear of 'loss of control' during labour
  Fear of fetal abnormality, still birth and neonatal death
  Preoccupation with desired sex of baby
  Reduced sexual activity; fears of loss of partner
  Concern about recurrence of postnatal depression
  Anxiety about parenting capacity

Table 1.2 Negative aspects of pregnancy

other times, for emotional as well as domestic and financial
security. It has also been shown that women are more sensitive
at this time to adverse life events such as health problems,
losses, crises or domestic difficulties.

Anxieties about the normality of the pregnancy will be
increased if there have been previous pregnancy disasters, if
there is a family history of birth trauma or abnormality, or if
there is doubt about the results of any of the antenatal predictive tests. Concern about the baby's size on the scan, persistent
vaginal bleeding, or raised blood pressure will affect psycho-

logical well-being and cause anxiety, self-blame and even resentment towards the fetus.

Prospective studies have shown that women who have frequent doubts about their ability to handle the demands of pregnancy and parenthood exhibit the most severe depressive symptoms in pregnancy. However, this may have a positive effect postpartum, as the woman 'rehearses' antenatally some of the negative aspects of motherhood. Other contributory personality factors may include over-dependency on partner or parents, and an over-sensitive, anxious or pessimistic personality.

Depression may accompany all physical symptoms, and the minor physical problems of pregnancy, such as nausea, heartburn, varicose veins and backache, will contribute to a lowering of mood. Of particular importance for emotional well-being is the reduction of Stage IV (the deepest level) sleep which occurs commonly in late pregnancy[12].

There is little factual information about the direct effect of the changed hormone levels in pregnancy on mood. It is thought that raised oestrogen levels give rise to nausea and emotional lability, whilst increased progesterone may cause sedation and lethargy. Thyroid hormone levels are raised in pregnancy[13] and may contribute to anxiety symptoms; raised cortisol levels, which also occur in pregnancy, are also known to correlate with depression.

Treatment of Psychological Problems in Pregnancy

Very simple interventions can often be most helpful in improving depressed mood or anxiety. The first requirement is to listen and to validate the feelings of the pregnant woman by giving her time and attention.

Practical Intervention

Simple advice-giving about having sufficient rest, particularly in the later stages of pregnancy, and avoiding major life changes, can be useful. The health visitor and the general practitioner are in an ideal position to identify antenatal anxieties and to offer reassurance and support. Women new to the area are particularly vulnerable; they lack a support network, and they may benefit from being introduced to other mothers at prenatal classes or mother and toddler groups.

Social workers can provide help with financial matters, and support for housing applications. They can also recommend the provision of practical support in terms of home help, or attendance at Social Services' family centres. Playgroups or child-minding for older children can provide welcome relief, particularly for the socially disadvantaged mother.

Psychotherapy

Where there are more specific psychological issues to be addressed, counselling or psychotherapy can be of benefit. This can be on an individual basis, or can also include the partner. Group therapy is less suitable because of the inevitable exit from the group at delivery, although mothers in a postnatal support group will often continue to attend through a subsequent pregnancy.

Some therapists are reluctant to embark on analytical psychotherapy during pregnancy because of the many 'real-life' changes going on at the same time, but some find it more advantageous because the women are highly motivated, and have a sense of urgency to change before the birth.

Brief cognitive behavioural therapy may be both more practical and acceptable than analytical psychotherapy.

Behavioural psychotherapy has a place in the treatment of antenatal agoraphobic or obsessive/compulsive symptoms, and may be effective in preventing a postnatal exacerbation.

Training in deep relaxation or auto-hypnosis can be helpful in the management of hyperemesis, allowing the woman to feel 'in charge' of her symptoms rather than at their mercy.

Community psychiatric nurses are invaluable in providing many of these interventions in the mother's own home.

Medication

Medication is rarely indicated, and should certainly be avoided where the mother has particular concerns about the normality of the fetus. Every attempt should be made to avoid medication during the first trimester. Later in pregnancy, the risks of toxicity, teratogenicity and possible longer-term neurobehavioural effects on the infant have to be balanced against the degree of mental disturbance in the mother.

Small doses of beta-blockers are helpful for anxiety symptoms, as are mild sedatives such as promethazine 20 mg or temazepam 10 mg at night for sleep disturbance.

Tricyclic antidepressants are not known to be associated with congenital abnormalities, but long-term behavioural effects have been reported in animal studies[14]. If required, the medication should be avoided in the first trimester unless the mother was already taking it at conception, the dose should be kept as low as possible, and discontinued two weeks before delivery to avoid withdrawal effects in the baby (*see* Case Study 1.2).

In women with pre-existing psychotic illness, where continuing medication is needed, it is probably better to give depot medication which avoids the 'peaks and troughs' of serum levels occurring with oral drugs.

Lithium is a special case. Although the absolute incidence of congenital abnormalities is not higher than in the general population, cardiac abnormalities are over-represented[15]. The most usual advice is to stop medication well before conception. However, where the risk of manic-depressive relapse is high, it may be preferable to continue lithium throughout the pregnancy, arranging for a detailed scan at 16 weeks to detect the possibility of cardiac abnormality in the fetus. The dose may need adjustment for the expansion of plasma volume during pregnancy, and be reduced near the time of delivery to avoid toxic levels during the diuresis in the first postnatal week. The use of diuretics for hypertension may also increase the serum level, which should be checked more frequently than usual[16].

The paediatrician should always be informed about mothers who are taking psychotropic medication in late pregnancy in case of untoward effects on the neonate at delivery.

Special Situations

The Teenage Mother

A survey of 79 pregnant teenagers[17] revealed that only 22% had actively wanted to conceive; 35% had not wanted to, and the remainder 'did not mind' or 'had not thought about it'. Over half of the 17-year-olds were in the latter category. In those who had not used contraception it was social considerations rather than lack of knowledge that prevented them from doing so. Wanting sex to be spontaneous, fearing that parents would find out that they were sexually active, and difficulty in obtaining supplies were among the reasons quoted. Sex education and contraceptive advice alone is therefore insufficient to prevent unwelcome teenage pregnancies; counselling about relationships and responsibilities is also important, and could take place within school or in the general practitioner's surgery if the parents are unable or unwilling to discuss such matters.

Twenty per cent of all teenage pregnancies occur within one month of becoming sexually active, and 50% within six months of first intercourse. A large study in the USA[18] showed that 55% of all teenage conceptions result in birth, the remainder being terminated. Over 50% of women under 18 years have no antenatal care until the second trimester, and 2% have little or none throughout the whole pregnancy.

There is a higher incidence of pregnancy complications, especially pregnancy induced hypertension, and of assisted deliveries and perinatal mortality in the under 16 age group, even when antenatal care is adequate[19]; low birth weight babies and still births are twice as common.

Many adolescent girls have unreal expectations about the partner's reaction to the pregnancy. Far from her fantasy of bringing them closer, she may end up alone, unsupported and with problems with accommodation and finance. She may be less willing to attend antenatal classes, and if her family of origin is not helpful, she may need individual support and education from the midwife, health visitor or social worker. She will also need support and counselling in deciding about termination or adoption.

Sixty per cent of teenagers who give birth before the age of 17 will have a repeat pregnancy before the age of 19.

The Older Mother

There are as many reasons for having a baby late in life as there are older mothers. However, they can be broadly grouped into those who have delayed pregnancy for reasons connected with career prospects, those with previous fertility problems, and the unplanned 'menopausal' pregnancy[20].

The 'last chance' pregnancy of the career woman who finds herself in her late thirties with the option of a baby now or childlessness for ever is fraught with emotional loading. She may have ambivalent feelings about the pregnancy, and will usually be aware of the increased risk of fetal abnormality. There is often an idealized view of pregnancy, and minor physical limitations may be magnified. She may grieve for the degree of control that she has had over her life so far, and at the same time be determined to show that she can be as successful at motherhood as she was in her career.

Because she has been working, she may not have established the local social networks that other mothers have, and may only take maternity leave late in the pregnancy, giving herself little time to make the emotional transition from working woman to mother. It is even more important for these women to be part of an antenatal group, and to work through with the midwife some of the negative as well as the positive aspects of motherhood.

The woman with a previous history of infertility or repeated miscarriages may see herself as a 'failure', blaming herself and being unable to believe that this pregnancy will be successful. There is preliminary evidence that mothers aged over 35 and expecting their first babies show decreased levels of attachment to the fetus[20]. An older mother may well withhold bonding to protect herself from further disappointment, but she will also deny herself the pleasure of anticipation, and the necessary antenatal 'rehearsal' for the reality of motherhood.

Where the older mother already has teenage children, her daughters may be envious of the mother's ability to procreate when they themselves are discouraged from doing so. Adolescent children may be embarrassed for their peer group to know that their mother is still sexually active, and resentful of the change to the *status quo*. A good family relationship will resolve these issues, but, where there is a normal adolescent striving for individuality, this may even lead to older children leaving home prematurely (*see* Case Study 1.3).

The mother herself may have worries about how she will cope physically with the demands of motherhood yet again, but many feel rejuvenated and are excited about the prospect of being an even better mother, with increased maturity and coping skills.

The Immigrant Mother

There have been few studies of immigrant women and their emotional experiences of pregnancy and birth. However, intuition tells us that it must be difficult for them to adjust to the management of childbirth in the UK, especially when normal practices are in conflict with their own religious or ethnic traditions. Asian mothers, for example, usually give birth at home, do not expect the partner to be present, and are attended for the first 40 days postpartum by female relatives. During this time they do not carry out domestic chores, and are expected to remain within the home.

One study of Asian women in London[21] showed that they accepted the 'medicalization' of pregnancy , and were regular clinic attenders. Most of the husbands were present at the delivery, and the women appreciated this. There was more emphasis on the sex of the baby – pleasure at having a boy and disappointment with a girl – than in a comparable Caucasian group. Some felt isolated in the postnatal ward because of language problems, and some were unable to keep the seclusion rules postpartum because female relatives and friends were not available.

It is important to be aware of cultural and religious differences, and to ask mothers if they have any objections to routine antenatal practices. They may, for example, prefer to see a woman doctor in the clinic if one is available, and to have a female companion during labour.

The Anorexic or Bulimic Mother

Pregnancy during the active phase of anorexia is of course unusual because of the suppression of ovulation associated with the condition. However, there are many women who have had an adolescent eating disorder in the past, and then go on to start a family. Many of these will be concerned about their changing weight and shape, although perhaps less so in the later stages when pregnancy is more obvious (*see* Case Study 1.4). Many with anorexia have anxieties about the adult role, and sexuality in particular. They may feel shame and guilt about their changing shape announcing their sexual activity to the world at large.

A follow-up of women with previous anorexia[22] has shown that they were less likely to want children than a comparable control group, and they were older at the time of the first pregnancy. Twice as many low birth weight babies were born to the anorexic mothers, and the perinatal mortality rate was increased sixfold. Surprisingly, there was no difference in the proportion of mothers choosing to breast feed, nor in the length of time that lactation continued, but the previous anorexics reported 28% of the children to have had 'eating problems'.

Bulimic patients report anxiety about possible damage to the fetus from the eating disorder[23]. The condition appears to improve during pregnancy in the majority, and, in a quarter of the sample, pregnancy appeared to be 'curative'. Nevertheless, symptoms returned postpartum in over half the patients, and more than half expressed anxieties about their babies being overweight.

The Epileptic Mother

A woman with epilepsy contemplating pregnancy should have pre-pregnancy counselling about the many difficulties that she may encounter. She may be concerned about the effects of her drug regimen on the fetus, the risk of increasing numbers of fits during pregnancy, her ability to cope with the demands of mothering, and the genetic risks for the child. It is sensible to give folate supplements before conception.

There is an increased risk of epilepsy in the child of between 3% and 6%, depending on the nature of the mother's epilepsy and the level of the seizure threshold[24].

Most anti-epileptic drugs are potentially teratogenic. Phenytoin, for example, carries a two- to threefold increase in the rate of congenital malformations, particularly cleft lip and palate, and cardiac malformations. Neural tube defects may be associated with valproate, and growth retardation with carbamazepine. There is an increased perinatal mortality rate.

The frequency of fits is increased during pregnancy in 45% of women, perhaps as a result of increased plasma volume and lower drug levels. In the presence of hypertension and oedema, it is important to bear in mind the differential diagnosis of eclampsia.

A woman with epilepsy who wishes to embark on a pregnancy should ideally be on a single drug, with serum concentrations maintained within the optimum range and checked monthly. Extra care should be taken in labour when the serum anti-epileptic levels may fall. The drugs are excreted in breast milk, but rarely cause problems. Drowsiness in the infant is an indication for artificial feeding, at least on a trial basis.

Despite all of the above, most epileptic women negotiate pregnancy, childbirth and bringing up a family very happily and successfully.

The Alcoholic Mother

The alcohol consumption of young fertile women has increased over recent years, as has the incidence of alcohol dependency. There are severe hazards to the fetus from excessive alcohol consumption in the mother in the very early days of the pregnancy, and possibly even in the pre-conceptual period. The full blown picture of fetal alcohol syndrome, which includes pre-and postnatal growth retardation, facial deformities and impaired psychomotor development, is thankfully rare, but there are more common complications amongst mothers who drink moderate amounts of alcohol. A Swedish study[25] showed that women who took alcohol 'at least 4–5 times a month' had babies who were small for gestational age, weighed less, were shorter and had smaller head circumferences than a comparable control group. The incidence of congenital anomalies was also increased, and there was a trend towards a higher neonatal death rate, although there were no actual cases of fetal alcohol syndrome.

More importantly, the alcohol intake was not recorded in the antenatal notes. People in general are unreliable about reporting their alcohol intake, and women attending an antenatal clinic may be even more so, fearing criticism and rejection. Only a trusting relationship with the clinic staff will reveal the truth and allow suitable intervention.

Women are perhaps less likely than men to have a high alcohol intake as part of their social activities. More of them may use alcohol as 'self-medication' for anxiety, depression and stress. Unfortunately, although it may initially relieve anxiety, it is a cerebral depressant, leading to frank depression and sleep disturbance, and hence often an escalation of consumption. No attempt to encourage withdrawal will then be successful unless the underlying mental state and/or social pressures are addressed. Carers will need to be non-critical in order not to compound the woman's guilt and distress; praise and encouragement for her efforts will be more helpful. Counselling on an individual basis and practical support may be needed.

The Management of Drug Abuse in Pregnancy

The number of pregnant women dependent on narcotic drugs has increased over recent years, and may be a real problem, particularly in inner city practices. Apart from the direct problems of drug abuse, these women often have multiple social difficulties including poverty, unsuitable accommodation and lack of social support. They are at higher risk of physical complications; obstetric complications, particularly placental abruption, are more common. They may also have had previous psychiatric illness. Almost all have a profound mistrust of authority figures, avoiding clinic attendance, and failing to co-operate with treatment programmes. Nevertheless, there are a significant number who will welcome the pregnancy as a time for change.

It is crucial to a successful outcome to build up an atmosphere of trust with the client, and to be uncritical and supportive. All those involved should have a coherent and carefully worked out plan for drug withdrawal; regular meetings between drug counsellors, general practitioners and social workers will minimize the risk of manipulation by the client[26]. One way of ensuring clinic attendance is to issue methadone prescriptions at the antenatal clinic, together with regular urine tests to screen for illicit drugs. A gradually reducing dose is given, attempting to stop medication altogether before delivery.

HIV testing after suitable counselling is advisable. Midwives should familiarize themselves with guidelines on the management of the HIV positive pregnant woman[27].

Follow-up on opiate addicted women postpartum shows that nearly 50% resume their drug habit after delivery, and that those who do are more likely to have the baby placed in the care of others[28].

Implications for Antenatal Care

Women themselves have very clear ideas of the kind of maternity care they would prefer. Sadly, many are frustrated and discontented with the care they receive. Long waiting times in hospital antenatal clinics appear to be the norm, and the consultations are often rushed and impersonal. Women may see a different doctor or midwife on each occasion, and often report a feeling as if they are 'on a conveyor belt'. Working women, in particular, complain about the length of time away from work for routine checks. In all comparisons in a large postal survey[29] attendance at general practitioner clinics was more appreciated. More women felt that waiting times were more acceptable, that they were given adequate information, and were able to ask sufficient questions.

So how can this general dissatisfaction be improved?

Individuality

Above all, it has to be remembered that each pregnancy has its own particular meaning for the individual woman at this particular time in her life. Pregnancy and birth are major life events, not just medical procedures. Adequate time for each woman to be treated as an individual in the antenatal clinic would be a beginning. Shifting the emphasis on physical health to include questions about the mother's emotional well-being is a vital part of good antenatal care.

Flexibility of Care

Flexibility of appointment times would also be of benefit. There might even be a good case for evening clinics for women who work or who have other young children and no available child-minder. Other specialties such as dentistry and genito-urinary medicine already follow this pattern. If we really value good antenatal care, and are really concerned about the mother as a person, it would be worth the inconvenience to staff.

Continuity of Care

Women say how much they appreciate continuity of care from the family doctor. They can also develop a good relationship with a community midwife, but this is less easy in the consultant unit setting. Some maternity units have set up a system of working in teams, in which each member of the team rotates duties between the antenatal clinic, the labour ward and the postnatal ward. Thus each individual woman is more likely to encounter a familiar face when she is admitted for delivery. This system also makes for better communication within the team about particularly anxious or sensitive mothers. Another alternative would be sectorization, with smaller teams working in designated parts of the catchment area.

Antenatal Education

The main aim of antenatal classes is to increase confidence in women, but surprisingly there has been little evaluation of this cost and time consuming programme. There is some evidence that the classes are predominantly attended by more middle-class than working-class mothers, and that the latter show a greater 'drop-out' rate.

It has been shown that the women reporting most benefit from antenatal classes are those who have a positive attitude to medical care in general[30], so that a sensitive approach from professionals in primary care is very important for its 'knock-on' effect. The same study has shown that there was a considerable increase in knowledge after the classes, but there was no correlation between knowledge level and satisfaction with outcome; attitudes reflecting confidence in health professionals and hospital care were more relevant. Another similar study found that confidence increased with time and anxiety levels fell[31]. Neither of these studies had control groups, so it is not possible to attribute the changes solely to the classes.

There was thought to be an additional benefit from local, community based classes, which created friendships and social support. It is certainly possible that more mothers from a wider range of social class might attend evening meetings, or daytime classes where a crèche is provided.

Dealing with Negative Aspects

Women often say that antenatal classes do not include time for the expression of negative feelings, such as anxieties about the normality of the baby, still birth and their own physical integrity. They have concerns about being cut, stretched or torn, and perhaps whether their husbands' feelings will change after the birth. They question their own capacity for maternal feelings, and wonder if they are really mature enough to care for a child. If a mother is not able to put into practice all that she has been taught, will the staff react with impatience; will she herself feel a 'failure' if she needs an assisted delivery? All of these are real and acceptable fears, not morbid or mistrustful, and should be allowed free ventilation during the pregnancy.

It may be that midwives and health visitors are unwilling to look at these issues themselves because of their own fears, or because they are concerned to instil confidence in their clients. It is important that professionals are aware of their own feelings, and prevent them from intruding in this situation.

Many women with postpartum emotional problems complain that they were not given sufficient information during the pregnancy about the risk and symptoms of postnatal depression. Midwives and health visitors, on the other hand, insist that they do so, but the mothers 'block out' what they say, not wanting to accept any negative information. The truth probably lies somewhere between these extremes.

In an attempt to overcome this communication problem, a single page information sheet has been prepared, and is included at the end of this chapter (*see* Appendix 1.1). It should be given not less than four weeks before delivery, to be kept with the co-operation card and referred to at a later date if need be. It has deliberately been kept brief and non-threatening, but should help women in doubt about their reactions. It also suggests helpful interventions, and gives details of self-help organizations.

And Finally...

Mothers need nurturing in order to be able to nurture. If the family or partner is not able to offer this, it is even more important that the professionals involved include this nurturing aspect within the framework of 'whole person' antenatal care.

Case Study 1.1

A patient who experienced severe postnatal depression wrote an account of her pregnancy as follows:

> 'During the pregnancy I was physically very well, playing hockey up to the 5th month. At that stage, I was affected by what was described as a 'hormone imbalance' and had a total change of personality. Instead of my normal extrovert self, I became clinging and dependent on my husband and family. I could not bear to be on my own for any length of time, and wept frequently. Life seemed to have no point, and had I not felt a deep moral responsibility for my unborn child, I would not have cared whether I lived or died.'

She made a full recovery following treatment for her postpartum depressive illness.

Case Study 1.2

A 30-year-old nurse married to a much older husband had had a salpingo-oophorectomy some years previously for an ectopic pregnancy. The early stages of her pregnancy were complicated by severe abdominal pain. Eventually an exploratory laparotomy was performed, and her appendix with adherent ovary and fallopian tube was removed. She was thus pregnant with no possibility of any future natural pregnancy, and her severe abdominal pain persisted after the operation. She was very pessimistic about a successful outcome of the pregnancy, constantly checking for fetal movements, and having recurrent nightmares about death.

She was encouraged to ventilate her ambivalent feelings about the pregnancy. Small doses of amitriptyline helped her poor sleep pattern and raised her pain threshold. A healthy boy was delivered at 38 weeks by caesarian section. She is currently pregnant again with a GIFT pregnancy.

Case Study 1.3

Joan was a woman in her mid-thirties who was pregnant for the third time. She had had her first baby at the age of 17, and, although the current pregnancy was unplanned, she was excited and pleased, especially to find that she was not the only older mother in the clinic. She looked forward to the baby in a way that she had not been able to when so much younger; there were now no financial difficulties, and she felt more emotionally stable. However, her daughter had reacted with shocked disbelief, and went to live with her boy-friend against her parents' wishes.

Joan's blood pressure rose towards the end of pregnancy and she was admitted for rest. Whilst in hospital, her daughter told her that she, too, was pregnant, and had decided to have a termination. Joan supported her daughter throughout the termination in the same hospital and visited her in the adjoining ward. Both mother and daughter felt confused about their feelings. They cried together about the 'lost' pregnancy, but were eventually able to share in the pleasure of the new baby in the family.

Case Study 1.4

Brenda was a 36-year-old woman with two children aged five and three from a previous marriage. She had just entered into a new relationship with a much younger man, and was 28 weeks pregnant when first referred. She had been uncharacteristically tearful and irritable for the previous three months. During the consultation, it emerged that she had been anorexic in her teens, and her current anxieties centred on her loss of attractiveness related her changing shape and the minor physical disabilities of pregnancy, and hence the possible loss of her new partner. She wore a T-shirt bearing the slogan: 'I'm not fat – just pregnant!'

A single counselling session helped her to confide in her husband who was able to reassure her that he was delighted about the baby, and found her even more attractive in her pregnant state.

Appendix 1.1

What is Postnatal Illness?

Postnatal illness (PNI) affects over 10% of all new mothers, sometimes beginning soon after the birth of the baby, sometimes weeks or months later. The symptoms can vary greatly in type, severity and duration. They can include tearfulness and deep despondency, together with profound exhaustion and often a feeling of not being able to cope with the baby. Mothers sometimes feel that they want to run away from the situation they are in, or at least have a short break from caring for the family. Irritability and tension, over-anxiety about their own or their baby's health may also occur. Many women feel extremely guilty about feeling so bad when they have a healthy baby, a nice house, and a helpful partner.

The good news is that PNI does not last for ever, even though women experiencing it find it hard to believe that they will ever recover. It does respond to treatment, often quite quickly, and life with a baby can be enjoyable again.

How to Help Yourself

- Share your feelings; don't bottle them up. Talk to your partner, mother, sister or a good friend. You will be surprised at how often you find others who have had a similar experience, and have recovered.

- Take as much rest as you can when you get home with the baby. Others are often willing to help in the early stages, but less so later if you have rejected them previously. Let friends know that you would like a quiet time each day, perhaps with no visitors at certain hours, and with the phone off the hook during these times.

- Don't try to be 'supermum' and do everything as before. Establish a comfortable routine in which meals are kept simple and housework is kept to a minimum.

- Do ask for help when you need it, not when everything has got on top of you.

- Take some time to care for yourself, perhaps to have a bath in peace, or to read. Some women find benefit from relaxation, and some from gentle exercise.

- Do try to get out of the house in the daytime, or invite friends in for tea. Motherhood alone can be lonely.

- If you feel that you have the symptoms of PNI, do get in touch with your midwife, health visitor or general practitioner. There are effective treatments available, and there is no virtue in suffering in silence.

Useful Contact Addresses

Meet-a-Mum Association
MAMA aims to help mothers make friends and give support, and overcome feelings of isolation and loneliness. They offer one-to-one contact, coffee mornings and social events to help mums who are lonely or depressed.
Telephone: 081 656 7318

The Association for Post-Natal Illness
APNI has telephone contacts for mothers with postnatal illness, usually with recovered mothers.
Telephone: 071 386 0868

Crysis
A self-help group dealing with persistently crying and sleepless babies.
Telephone: 071 404 5011

National Childbirth Trust
NCT provide friendship and support for parents and families, and have local breast-feeding counsellors.
Telephone: 081 992 8637

Homestart
This organization provides practical and emotional help for the
mothers of children under the age of five. There are branches in
many, but not all, areas.
Telephone: 0533 554988

Twins and Multiple Births Association
Telephone 051 348 0020

References

1. Giel R and Kidd C. (1965) Some observations on pregnancy in the unmarried student. *British Journal of Psychiatry*. **111**: 591–4.

2. Raphael-Leff J. (1990) Psychotherapy and pregnancy. *Journal of Reproductive and Infant Psychology*. **8**: 119–35.

3. Kumar R and Robson KM. (1984) A prospective study of emotional disorders in childbearing women. *British Journal of Psychiatry*. **144**: 35–47.

4. Hrasky M and Morice R. (1986) The identification of psychiatric disturbance in an obstetric and gynaecological population. *Australian and New Zealand Journal of Psychiatry*. **20**: 63–9.

5. Sharp DJ. (1988) Validation of the 30-item GHQ in early pregnancy. *Psychological Medicine*. **18**: 503–7.

6. Powers PS, Johnson T, Knuppel R, *et al.* (1986) Psychiatric disorders in high-risk pregnancy. *Comprehensive Psychiatry*. **27**: 159–64.

7. Poland ML, Giblin PT, Lucas CP, *et al.* (1986) Psychobiological determinants of pregnancy-induced hypertension. *Journal of Psychosomatic Obstetrics and Gynaecology*. **5**: 85–92.

8. Out JJ, Vierhout ME, Verhage F, *et al.* (1986) Characteristics and motives of women choosing elective induction of labour. *Journal of Psychosomatic Research*. **30**: 375–80.

9. Berkowitz GS and Kasl SV. (1983) The role of psychosocial factors in spontaneous pre-term delivery. *Journal of Psychosomatic Research*. **27**: 283–90.

10. Welles-Nystrom BL and de Chateau P. (1987) Maternal age and transition to motherhood. *Acta Psychiatrica Scandinavica*. **76**: 719–25.

11. Appleby L. (1991) Suicide during pregnancy and the first postnatal year. *British Medical Journal*. **302**: 137–40.

12. Karacan I, Williams RL, Hursch CJ, *et al.* (1969) Some implications of the sleep pattern of late pregnancy for post-partum emotional disturbances. *British Journal of Psychiatry.* **115**: 929–35.

13. Rodin A and Rodin A. (1989) Thyroid disease in pregnancy. *British Journal of Hospital Medicine.* **41**: 234–41.

14. Kerns LL. (1986) Treatment of mental disorders during pregnancy. A review of psychotropic drug risks and benefits. *Journal of Nervous and Mental Disease.* **174**: 652–8.

15. Robinson GE, Stewart DE and Flak E. (1986) The rational use of psychotropic drugs in pregnancy and post-partum. *Canadian Journal of Psychiatry.* **31**: 183–90.

16. Schou M. (1990) Lithium treatment during pregnancy, delivery and lactation: An update. *Journal of Clinical Psychiatry.* **51**: 410–3.

17. Phoenix A. (1989) Influences on previous contraceptive use/non-use in pregnant 16–19 year olds. *Journal of Reproductive and Infant Psychology.* **7**: 211–25.

18. Hechtman L. (1989) Teenage mothers and their children: Risks and problems: A review. *Canadian Journal of Psychiatry.* **34**: 569–75.

19. McGrew MC and Shore WB. (1991) The problem of teenage pregnancy. *Journal of Family Practice.* **32**: 17–25.

20. Berryman JC and Windridge KC. (1993) Pregnancy after 35: A preliminary report on maternal-foetal attachment. *Journal of Reproductive and Infant Psychology.* **11**: 169–73.

21. Woollett A and Dosanjh-Matwala N. (1990) Asian women's experience of childbirth in East London: The support of fathers and female relatives. *Journal of Reproductive and Infant Psychology.* **8**: 11–22.

22. Brinch M, Isager T and Tolstrup K. (1988) Anorexia nervosa and motherhood: Reproductional pattern and mothering behaviour of 50 women. *Acta Psychiatrica Scandinavica.* **77**: 98–104.

23. Lacey JH and Smith G. (1987) Bulimia nervosa: The impact of pregnancy on mother and baby. *British Journal of Psychiatry.* **150**: 777–81.

24. Espir MLE. (1986) Epilepsy and pregnancy. *Update.* **32**: 703–8.

25. Hollstedt C, Dahlgren L and Rydberg U. (1983) Outcome of pregnancy in women treated at an alcohol clinic. *Acta Psychiatrica Scandinavica*. **67**: 236–48.

26. Riley D. (1987) The management of the pregnant drug addict. *Bulletin of the Royal College of Psychiatrists*. **11**: 362–4.

27. Forbes PB. (1986) The significance of AIDS in obstetric practice. *British Journal of Hospital Medicine*. **35**: 342–6.

28. Fraser AC and Cavanagh S. (1991) Pregnancy and drug addiction: Long term consequences. *Journal of the Royal Society of Medicine*. **84**: 530–2.

29. Taylor A. (1986) Maternity services: The consumer's view. *Journal of the Royal College of General Practitioners*. **36**: 157–60.

30. Rutter DR, Quine L and Hayward R. (1988) Satisfaction with maternity care: Psychosocial factors in pregnancy outcome. *Journal of Reproductive and Infant Psychology*. **6**: 261–9.

31. Astbury J. (1980) The crisis of childbirth: Can information and childbirth education help? *Journal of Psychosomatic Research*. **24**: 9.

2 Labour

Women approach labour with a variety of emotions ranging from 'confident' to 'terrified', determined largely by the attitudes and feelings they bring to the experience. Whatever these may be, birth is invested with an intensity of feeling rarely experienced at other times. It is an experience which is recollected throughout life, sometimes in the most amazing detail. All women hope that it will be a fulfilling and life-enhancing experience, and most will be fearful of their own ability to match its importance with their own coping skills.

The Place of Birth

Most deliveries now take place in hospital, and many women who would prefer a home birth are denied it. Comparisons of safety are hard to make, since there is a selection procedure; only low risk women are permitted to deliver at home. The Dutch experience[1] has shown that the perinatal mortality rate of hospital births is five times that of home confinements, and a Welsh study has found the postnatal depression rate to be three times greater in patients who have had hospital deliveries[2].

Most hospitals have made compromises towards women's wishes by providing a 'birthing room', which is less clinical than the traditional labour ward, and allowing women to have some choice in their birth plan, including early discharge. Baths, enemas and shaving are no longer routine. There is thankfully now more choice about birth position, although the dreaded lithotomy stirrups are still in use during forceps deliveries and perineal stitching. In spite of these practical concessions, the appreciation of emotional factors during labour seems sometimes to have changed more slowly.

Dignity and privacy are part of proper self-worth, and both

are in jeopardy when entering any hospital situation. This is not appreciated enough by those who work in hospitals, because of their own familiarity with the surroundings and procedures. A woman entering hospital is separated from her own surroundings and from the external aspects of her own identity, her clothes and belongings. She may have intimate questions asked within earshot of others, be addressed in terms more appropriate to a nursery school child, and expose her 'private' parts to anyone who happens to enter the labour room.

It goes without saying that women should be treated as responsible, competent adults. Attendants should not address them by Christian name unless invited to do so, and anonymous terms of endearment should be avoided. Addressing the woman as 'mother' also implies that the carer cannot be bothered to remember her name. No-one should approach the labour room without knocking on the door first, and no-one should enter until invited to do so. Anyone who does enter should have a good reason to be there, and should immediately be introduced to the mother by name and description of role, such as: 'Mrs Brown, this is Andrew Smith, the medical student who is attached to the labour ward this week. Are you happy for him to be present at the delivery?'

The Mother's Experience

Women in labour experience heightened awareness, and become acutely, and quite properly, self-absorbed. Thus, all sensations are magnified, and referred to themselves, leading to misinterpretation of events considered quite normal to the staff. Great care is needed to give slow and careful explanations to the mother, checking back with her that she has really understood. Many women report that professional staff talk to each other or to the partner rather than to herself, making her feel useless and incompetent. Labouring women seem to be particularly sensitive about 'feeling out of control', partly as a result of their own fears about internal control of both physical and emotional functions, but also because the use of technology can increase this feeling of being 'taken over' by machines.

Accelerated labour is a case in point, where women may feel that this is more for the convenience of the staff than for their own benefit, and the rate of the oxytocin drip, and hence their own pain and contraction rate, is totally under the control of the doctor or midwife.

A study which looked at women's reactions according to the degree of technology used in labour[3] found that fewer women in the high technology group enjoyed the birth or felt in control in labour, and that more of them were liable to be unhappy in the postnatal ward. Primiparous patients report the greatest discrepancy between their expectations of childbirth and the outcome, not because their expectations were too high, but because they had more unexpected obstetric interventions, such as assisted delivery. It is suggested that primiparous women, in particular, should be prepared for a wide range of obstetric interventions, and the reality that some of their expectations will not be met.

Labour is accepted as being painful in the majority of cases, but professionals may be less aware of the variety of other emotional factors which are also experienced. The percentages of women describing adverse symptoms in labour in a Norwegian study of hospital births[4] are shown in Table 2.1.

Symptom	%
Unhappiness in labour	87
Labour 'very difficult'	60
Losing track of time and place	50
Labour 'intolerably' painful	33
A feeling of not coping well	29
Extreme loss of control	26
Severe anxiety	22

Table 2.1 Adverse symptoms described during labour

A study of pain in labour[5] showed that recall assessed on the McGill Pain Questionnaire showed a wide variation of intensity, and was predictably higher in primiparous women. The mean level was higher than other patients who rated the pain of cancer or a phantom limb. The descriptions of the pain were vivid; it was described as 'cramping, aching, heavy, tight, tiring, intense and exhausting'.

Michel Odent[6] has also documented the very real fear of death experienced by many labouring women in a variety of settings throughout the world, both in the past and the present day. He associated this with rapid and efficient labour, postulating that the high adrenalin levels occurring in states of extreme fear have an oxytocic effect, leading to the 'fetus ejection reflex'. He also feels that it may be related to reduction of activity in the higher centres of the brain allowing disinhibition, and the expression of primitive fears. Most midwives will be aware of the disinhibited behaviour and language of some women during labour.

Helene Deutsch, a psychoanalyst, went so far as to write in 1924[7]: 'Childbirth is ... an orgy of masochistic pleasure for the female made even more exciting by the possibility of associated death.'

Few present day obstetricians or mothers would agree. However, it is not so long since these fears had real justification in terms of a substantial maternal mortality rate, and it is still true that healthy young women are probably 'nearer to death' during labour than they have been at any time since their own birth. Indeed, a recent study of 2 000 consecutive deliveries showed that a quarter of the women experienced some morbidity associated with pregnancy or labour, and 19 potentially life threatening episodes occurred[8]. These included fulminating pre-eclampsia, pulmonary embolus, uterine rupture and post-partum haemorrhage leading to hysterectomy.

We recognize the profound after effects of the fear of death or injury in those experiencing accidents, war, or natural disasters, but perhaps because childbirth is so common, we close our minds to the possibility of post-traumatic stress disorder in newly delivered women[9] (*see* Case Study 2.1).

The Professional Carers

Those attending women in labour hold a privileged position within the field of medicine. They are present at the climax of a nine-month period of anxiety and hope, at the moment when a couple becomes a family, and when the parents, the creators, come face to face with their creation.

A common complaint of unhappy mothers is of unsympathetic staff. Many midwives have not had children of their own, and male doctors will not have experienced labour at first hand. They may perhaps become 'immunized' to the distress and discomfort of labouring women as simply a part of their ordinary working day. Equally, their own anxiety about a slowly progressing labour, or having several women in labour at the same time, may make them appear irritable and impatient.

A woman suffering from postnatal depression wrote:

> 'My second labour had been "copybook" – no drugs, no stitches and no breast feeding problems. But I had been attended by three different midwives in the space of two hours, all of them rather off-hand, and I had met none of them before.'

It is even possible that some doctors and midwives feel envy of the labouring mother, to the extent that they have unconscious wishes to 'take over' both the birth (which of course they would have managed much better), and the baby (which of course would have been more perfect), making both their own[10]. These envious desires can affect the carer's ability to see the woman as a whole person, with a brain and a psyche as well as a uterus. To hand the baby to the parents, to see their enjoyment of each other, may be exquisitely painful for the attendant, and be associated with a real sense of loss unless these envious feelings are identified and resolved.

Midwife training has only within the past year become a continuous assessment, which includes attitudes to parents and communication skills as well as technical knowledge tested by examination. One tutor with 14 years' experience could not recall any student failing because of personality problems, but was able to recognize these problems in some of the qualified staff. After all, most midwives' first training is in general hospitals, where their function is to 'do things to' sick and helpless patients, and it is not always easy to make the transition to 'being with' healthy, competent women.

Another important issue is the feelings that mothers project on to the midwife or doctor, depending on their previous experience with authority figures, the parents in particular (*see* Case Study 2.2). Women with domineering mothers may fear the same approach from the midwife; women with ineffectual mothers and caring fathers may invest their confidence in a male doctor, and see the midwife as inadequate. The midwife is truly in a dilemma, which is to care for a mother whom she may only just have met, at a deeply personal level, yet not to take personally any angry or hostile feelings the mother may express.

'Debriefing' is an important part of the care given to a mother after labour is complete. She will undoubtedly do this with friends and family over and over again, and her description of events will be coloured by the emotions which accompanied them. It is helpful on two counts to do this with the professional who has delivered her, soon after the birth. Firstly, misconceptions can be put right; explanations can be given about why pain relief was given or withheld at a particular time, and why it was not the mother's 'incompetence' that led to an instrumental delivery. Secondly, it is an important learning experience for the carer to know how the labour was experienced by the mother. This can help the carer to understand that what was said or done was not always interpreted in the way it was meant. Carers can then modify their own approaches to women in labour, in order to be more sensitive to their needs.

Lest there be any doubt about the importance of the midwife's role, there is a significant correlation between women's perception of unmet needs in relation to the midwife and depressed mood on the fifth postpartum day[4]. Mothers consistently relate the midwife's sensitivity to their needs as the most important aspect of care in labour, and see this as more important than her professional competence.

The interactions which occur at the time of delivery are indelibly printed on the mother's mind, and it is possible that the amnesia for the event which some women demonstrate is nothing more than an unconscious denial in cases where these interactions are unsatisfactory. Most family doctors are aware of a closer, freer relationship with women they have delivered. This time is a 'critical period' in a technical as well as a real sense, and can engender mutual respect and trust. Likewise, if mishandled, dislike and mistrust may smoulder and lead to difficulties with future deliveries, or, more likely, provide the content, if not the impetus, for the development of postnatal depression.

The Partner's Role

It is now commonplace for fathers to be present at the birth, and this is generally thought to be good practice. However, not all partners are equally helpful, and some may have anxieties about their ability to cope. There has been little evaluation of the benefits, and there is conflicting evidence about the effect of fathers' presence on pain levels. One study showed that most mothers appreciated the involvement of the partner, and, where his presence was experienced as helpful, there was a subjective assessment of lower levels of pain[11]. However, objectively, there was no difference in the use of analgesia by these women.

Some women report that the partners seemed more interested in the technology than in the labour itself. This may be a defence mechanism in fathers to divert their own attention from the experience of seeing the woman in pain, and feeling helpless. Technology they understand, emotions perhaps less so. It certainly appears that fathers' emotional involvement with the pregnancy mitigates their own anxiety, and that active involvement decreases the incidence of physical symptoms in fathers[12].

Women often complain if the baby is first handed to the father. However exhausted or apparently disinterested the mother appears to be, and even if she needs help and encouragement to hold the baby, this is never good practice, and can lead to later regret and difficulties with attachment.

Where the baby's father is absent, or unwilling to be present, most women will opt for a close friend or relative to take his place. In other settings, the presence of a professional companion, a 'doula', has been shown to reduce the length and complications of labour[13,14].

Case Study 2.1

Julia had her first baby three months before referral by her family doctor. Her complaints were of low mood and severe anxiety about possible physical problems in herself and her child.

She described numerous difficulties with the pregnancy and delivery, including mislaid blood test results and delayed procedures. She was unhappy about a sudden and unexplained change in anaesthetic procedure at delivery, and experienced extreme pain. On complaining to the doctor, she felt that she was being blamed for having a low pain tolerance. She also required a blood transfusion and later felt that the postnatal ward staff were neither helpful nor understanding.

She was discharged early from the postnatal ward at her own request, and described feeling 'bitter' about the entire delivery. She felt that it was all made worse by inadequate explanations of the procedures to which she was subjected, and lack of support from her husband and in-laws. She felt vulnerable, lonely, and scared of future pregnancies.

Julia had had a difficult childhood, with a violent and unpredictable father who suffered from depressive mood swings. She recalled that she and her mother often fled to friends when his aggression got out of hand, and that she was afraid to sleep when her parents were arguing.

Ventilation of her feelings was helpful, and she began to understand that her fear and mistrust of authority figures stemmed from her childhood fears of her father's unpredictable aggression. She agreed that she had seen the female role as 'passive' and 'doomed to suffer'. Julia began to see that her own husband could be trusted to support her and the baby, and her depressed mood resolved without medication.

Case Study 2.2

Karen presented three months postpartum with severe panic attacks and inability to be left alone with the baby. She constantly telephoned her husband at work for reassurance, and felt that she was burdening friends by continually asking for support.

This was a very unusual state for her to be in. She had previously worked as a senior and extremely competent psychiatric nurse, often caring for mothers with postnatal illness. She blamed herself for her 'inadequacy and incompetence' as a mother, and had developed secondary depressive symptoms.

Karen's pregnancy had been complicated by severe pregnancy-induced hypertension necessitating frequent hospital admissions. Labour had been induced at 36 weeks, and progressed slowly but painfully. Her blood pressure continued to rise during labour, and she was aware of anxiety from the staff about possible eclampsia. She thought that, because of her nursing background, they did not wish to worry her unduly, but she felt angry when they talked to her partner rather than to herself.

At one point she had a severe headache, and remembered panic in the labour room, and someone shouting for the 'crash' team. On regaining consciousness, she was told that she had had a healthy baby girl by emergency caesarian section. However, the baby was in special care for a few days, and bonding was slow to take place.

She was able to understand that her normal feelings of competence and control had been severely dented by her experience. She had temporarily 'lost faith' in her physical and emotional integrity, but renewed confidence built up over a period of weeks following brief psychotherapy.

References

1. Kloosterman GJ. (1982) The universal aspects of childbirth: Human birth as a socio-psychosomatic paradigm. *Journal of Psychosomatic Obstetrics and Gynaecology.* 1: 35–41.

2. Robinson J. (1975) How hospitals alienate mothers. *Mind Out.* (March/April): 7–9.

3. Booth CL and Meltzoff AN. (1984) Expected and actual experience in labour and delivery and their relationship to maternal attachment. *Journal of Reproductive and Infant Psychology.* 2: 79–91.

4. Thune Larsen K-B and Moller-Pedersen K. (1988) Childbirth experience and post-partum emotional disturbance. *Journal of Reproductive and Infant Psychology.* 6: 229–40.

5. Niven C and Gijsbers K. (1984) Obstetric and non-obstetric factors related to labour pain. *Journal of Reproductive and Infant Psychology.* 2: 61–78.

6. Odent MR. (1991) Fear of death during labour. *Journal of Reproductive and Infant Psychology.* 9: 43–7.

7. Deutsch H. (1924) Psychoanalysis of the sexual function of women. Ed: Roazen P. (1991) Publ. H. Karnac.

8. Stones W, Lim W, Al-Azzawi F, *et al.* (1991) An investigation of maternal morbidity with identification of life-threatening 'near-miss' episodes. *Health Trends.* 23: 13–5.

9. Bloor RN and Jones RA. Post-traumatic stress disorder and sexual function. *British Journal of Sexual Medicine.* 15: 170–2.

10. Dean M. (1978) Home sweet hospital. *World Medicine.* 13: 21–6.

11. Niven C. (1985) How helpful is the presence of the husband at childbirth? *Journal of Reproductive and Infant Psychology.* 3: 45–53.

12. Teichman Y and Lahav Y. (1987) Expectant fathers: Emotional reactions, physical symptoms and coping styles. *British Journal of Medical Psychology.* 60: 225–32.

13. Klaus M, *et al.* (1986) Effects of social support in parturition on maternal and infant morbidity. *British Medical Journal.* **293**: 585–8.

14. Chalmers B and Wolman W. (1993) Social support in labour: A selective review. *Journal of Psychosomatic Obstetrics and Gynaecology.* **14**: 1–15.

3   The Early Puerperium

Normal Changes

The emotional changes taking place in the first few days after childbirth, particularly with a first baby, are probably greater than at any other time in a woman's life. Some of the positive and negative changes to be expected are detailed below. Feelings may oscillate wildly between the two extremes, or even coexist, creating a true ambivalence. This makes it difficult for the mother, and certainly her carers, to establish a steady foundation for all the new experiences and learning she will have to assimilate in the following days and weeks.

Positive changes may be:

- elation
- satisfaction
- increased closeness to partner
- closeness to, and identification with, her own mother
- gradual 'falling in love' with the baby
- protectiveness towards the infant
- change in marital relationship: now 'mother and father' not 'husband and wife'.

Negative changes may be:

- distress or disappointment about the delivery
- anxiety about the baby, especially if in special care
- rejection of or ambivalence towards the infant
- doubts about her own ability to cope with motherhood

- fears of harming the baby: anxieties about being alone with the child

- resentment of baby being the centre of attention

- feeling of 'emptiness'

- anxiety about physical damage during the birth

- identification with her own mother: anxieties if the relationship was not good in childhood

- overwhelming sense of responsibility

- resentment at loss of freedom

- physical discomfort.

The mother's adjustment in this critical period will depend on many factors: her experience of the delivery, her experience of being mothered herself, her relationship with the baby's father and his ability to be supportive and understanding, her own personality and degree of maturity, and her expectations of motherhood, both positive and negative.

It will also depend a good deal on the kind of care she receives from her professional attendants. If they are sensitive to her mood, her anxieties and her needs, and encouraging towards her developing maternal skills, she will negotiate this difficult period more easily, becoming confident and happy.

The new mother will need to establish her own relationship with her baby, and will need privacy and uninterrupted time to explore its body, to establish eye contact, and to 'learn its language'. No advice from books or professionals can replace the mother's own ability to interpret the small movements, gestures, vocalizations and expressions of her own child. In fact, too much, or conflicting, advice has been found to impair the mother's confidence in her own decision making.

The realization of the responsibility of a baby is often overwhelming at first, and most women will have times of doubt about whether they are truly capable of accepting such dependency, and the need to put someone else's needs before their own, for the rest of their lives. There is also the anxiety of 'sharing' herself between this dependent creature and her partner, or with the other children in the family. She may worry whether she has enough love left for this new arrival, or enough energy and time to sustain adult relationships as well.

Thus each woman's response will be individual, even idiosyncratic, and changeable from day to day, or even hour to hour. Yet the surroundings and culture on the postnatal ward are necessarily regimented to a greater or lesser degree, depending on staffing levels and the sensitivity of the staff involved. In a consumer survey of postnatal care a mother commented[1]: 'During labour the care I received was fantastic ... but after the birth I felt that you were left to get on with it ... the baby didn't seem important in their scheme of things.'

The same study showed that 46% of women felt that they had insufficient sleep, and 22% of mothers felt depressed 'for most of the time' when they had their babies in hospital consultant units.

A large survey of mothers delivered in hospital[2] revealed that the midwives had difficulty in interpreting signs of emotional distress in mothers. For example, they reported that only 1% of the mothers had experienced the 'blues', whilst also noting that over 20% had been tearful, and 15% had experienced sleep disturbance. The tendency appeared to be for midwives to attribute these symptoms to physical discomfort or difficulties with feeding, or alternatively to see some degree of emotional distress as 'normal', and therefore to be ignored. Both the staff doctors and the midwives appeared to use physical criteria to assess whether the mother was fit for discharge, paying little attention to her level of confidence, emotional state or the level of care available within the home.

One group of women were given a 'technology score' related to the degree of intervention during labour[3]. Three times as many of the high scoring group reported themselves as depressed postpartum in hospital. Another relevant factor was the number of children already in the family.

Especially in the present trend towards early discharge, women pass through the postnatal ward so quickly that it is difficult for midwives to get to know them at a personal level. However, physical issues, for example blood loss, the height of the fundus, and perineal healing, are 'checked off' daily until they are satisfactory. It might be equally helpful to have a similar list of emotional adjustments.

- Does the mother feel that she is getting sufficient sleep?
- Does she feel that she is having sufficient rest during the day?
- Does she have a choice between rooming-in and having the baby in the nursery at night?
- Have her wishes about night feeds been respected?
- Does she feel that she has sufficient privacy?
- Is she happy with the hospital food?
- Is she confident about her chosen infant feeding pattern?
- Have any special religious or cultural needs been met?
- Has she any worries about the care of older children at home?
- Does she wish other children or grandparents to visit?
- What are her wishes about discharge from hospital?
- Does she have sufficient help at home to go back to?

The Postnatal 'Highs'

A degree of elation is entirely normal in the very early post-partum days, particularly if the labour went well, and if the partner and family are happy and congratulatory. It may be a surprise to learn that, in some, this elation is extreme; in about 16% of women is sufficiently marked to meet the diagnostic criteria for hypomania[4]. In these cases, the mother may be unusually cheerful, overactive, and overtalkative, with 'racing' thoughts and difficulty with concentration. This is sometimes associated with irritability, especially when others try to bring her back to reality. It appears to be self-limiting, and may be related to the dramatic fall in hormone levels within the first few postpartum days. An alternative explanation is that sleep loss, if the mother is delivered during the night or is having disturbed nights with the baby, can precipitate mild hypomanic symptoms in vulnerable women[5].

The 'Blues'

The sequel to this episode of elation may be a period of low or unstable mood – the 'blues' – occurring typically between the fourth and tenth day postpartum. This is very common, occurring in 50–70% of all newly delivered women whether they are primiparous or multiparous[6,7]. It is so common as to be a 'normal' occurrence, but it can be very upsetting to mothers, and often to staff, if they are unaware of the possibility.

It often follows on from a disturbed night's sleep, sometimes including frightening and vivid dreams, and even brief disorientation and hallucinatory experiences on waking. The predominant symptom is that of emotional over-reactivity. Mood may fluctuate from happy and laughing at one moment, to tearful and sad at the next. Trivial problems, for example with feeding, may provoke major reactions.

Anxiety is often an associated feature, commonly being focused on difficulties with breast-feeding, since the blues often coincides with the day of maximum milk production, when there is engorgement and discomfort. Extreme anxiety can lead to feelings of unreality and detachment. Confusion and forgetfulness is sometimes reported, and psychological testing has in fact shown some cognitive deficit and difficulty with abstract thought in the early days postpartum[8].

There may also be a degree of hostility, although this is rarely directed towards the baby. The 'blues' day is the one where the partner is liable to be harangued if he is late visiting, or if he brings the wrong clothes, and where the mother may be angry and irritable with the midwives, especially if they are thought to be giving contradictory advice.

Headache, often of a migrainous type, is common, occurring in about one-third of postnatal women, and being more common when there is a past history of migraine.

The timing of the maximum 'blues' score often correlates with the day of maximum diuresis and weight loss[9].

Several researchers[10,11,12] have attempted to devise a 'blues' questionnaire, the most recent of which is given at the end of the chapter (*see* Appendix 3.1). Most questionnaires are unsatisfactory in some respects, as it is almost impossible to quantify changeability of mood, or to include the multiplicity of symptoms which may occur. The syndrome is obvious enough to those who work with postnatal women, but it is helpful to have a standardized assessment procedure for research purposes.

Treatment of the 'Blues'

Thankfully, the condition is usually short-lasting, being only 24–48 hours in duration. Treatment is rarely required, but it is as well to avoid over-stimulation, restricting visitors, perhaps, and ensuring a good night's sleep the next night. If the symptoms are severe, mothers may need a good deal of reassurance that they are not 'going mad'.

There are distinct resemblances between the 'blues' and severe premenstrual symptoms, so that, if the female staff can empathize with the mother's feelings, they will be less likely to react adversely to her anger or distress.

Causes of the 'Blues'

Some of the psychosocial factors contributing to the 'blues' have been described above. However, the mother's personality, her experience of pregnancy, and her expectations surrounding the birth also have a significant part to play. Postnatal 'blues' has been shown to relate to anxiety in pregnancy, experiencing pregnancy as unpleasant, fear of childbirth, and the mother having an anxious or pessimistic personality. A more recent study has found it to be more common in women who have had a caesarian section, and whose babies were of low birth weight[13,14].

Another large study of Norwegian women[15] found that the factors most closely related to low mood on the fifth day were loss of control during labour, anxiety in the week before delivery, and 'unmet needs in relation to the midwife'. This implies that midwives have a crucial role to play in emotional well-being in the early puerperium.

The 'blues' seems to occur equally often in mothers in hospital and those discharged early, in primiparae and multiparae, and in breast-feeding and bottle-feeding mothers. It has been thought that it is simply a non-specific reaction to stress, similar to that which might occur after an operation. However, a careful study has shown that it is very different in symptom pattern, and also in its timing, in relation to the potentially stressful event[16,17].

Also in favour of a distinct aetiology and relationship to childbirth is the finding that it occurs almost equally in women from very different cultures, including Africa, Australia and Jamaica[18-20], although, in these settings, physical symptoms may predominate. The only study showing a cultural difference in incidence is one demonstrating a lower rate of occurrence in Japanese mothers[21]. It may be that they are less willing to 'lose face' by admitting to symptoms than are mothers in the West.

Although the 'blues' may be mild and transient in itself, it has two important implications. First, because of its timing within the first postpartum week, the symptoms can be misinterpreted as the early signs of a much more serious psychiatric illness, puerperal psychosis. Worse still, the early signs of psychosis can be attributed to 'just the blues', and not taken seriously enough. If there is a personal or family history of severe psychiatric illness, and the 'blues' appears to be severe, or unduly prolonged, a psychiatric opinion should be sought without delay.

Secondly, because the 'blues' is so frequent, because it occurs very soon after the dramatic postpartum hormone changes, and because it shares some characteristics with other psychiatric syndromes associated with hormonal imbalance, such as the premenstrual syndrome, it has been thought that it would be an ideal model for the investigation of the more severe postnatal illnesses. This has not unfortunately been the case; the evidence is confusing and often contradictory.

The Evidence for Hormonal Causation

We know that the hormonal changes occurring immediately after childbirth are both enormous and rapid, a phenomenon that occurs at no other time in a woman's life. In the face of this huge change, and the individual variation in hormonal pattern, it is not perhaps surprising that few significant differences in hormone levels have been found between subjects with the 'blues' and those without.

There is also no reason to suppose that hormone levels alone are causal. It may be that women differ in their susceptibility to the normal hormonal changes after delivery, depending on their genetic vulnerability or personality.

One of the earlier investigations revealed that there was no overall correlation of hormone levels with the 'blues' but that individual symptoms were related to separate hormonal changes. For example, sleeplessness was related to the degree of fall in oestrogen, and depressed mood weakly related to the fall in progesterone[22]. Other investigations since have been contradictory.

One study comparing hormone levels in saliva between women with and without the 'blues' showed that progesterone and oestradiol were significantly higher in the 'blues' subjects, but that cortisol levels were similar[23]. However, two more recent studies showed higher levels of serum cortisol associated with the blues[24,25]. This is similar to the high levels found in depression at other times.

Prolactin levels have been found to be higher in 'blues' subjects, and to correlate with anxiety and depression[26].

There is some evidence that thyroid hormone levels are increased during pregnancy, but most of the T_3 and T_4 is bound to thyroxine binding globulin and is therefore inactive. In some cases this is followed by a transient mild hypothyroidism postnatally. There is no evidence linking these factors to early onset emotional disorders.

Other researchers have thought that hormones may have an indirect effect through alternative biochemical pathways. For example, low levels of neurotransmitters in the brain are known to be associated with depressive illness. Serotonin, in particular, has been shown to be low in the blood of depressed patients and in the brains of suicides. One of the 'building blocks' for serotonin is tryptophan, an amino acid; tryptophan levels have been shown to be low in association with depressed mood on the sixth postpartum day[27]. Nevertheless, giving tryptophan supplements to postnatal women seemed not to prevent the 'blues', so that the relationship between the two is probably indirect, and must also depend on other factors[28]. A more recent study of serotonin in platelets has found a trend towards low levels in patients with 'blues' symptoms, and high levels in those who were elated[29].

There are also reported changes in α-2-adrenoceptor sites in platelets being generally lower postpartum than in the late stage of pregnancy, but higher in those women with 'blues' symptoms than in those without[30]. Similar high adrenoceptor sensitivity has been found in association with lower adrenergic activity and depression. This may be a secondary change in response to the drop in oestradiol and progesterone levels in the puerperium.

It is perhaps not surprising that a transient syndrome with such a diverse constellation of symptoms, and such a large psychosocial component to its aetiology, has not shown any clear hormonal or biochemical correlations. In the face of such enormous hormonal changes over just a few days, the wonder is that so many women adjust so well and so quickly.

Appendix 3.1

The Blues Questionnaire: Kennerley 1989[10]

Subject name: No:

Date: Days postpartum:

Below is a list of words which newly delivered mothers have used to describe how they are feeling. Please indicate HOW YOU HAVE BEEN FEELING TODAY by ticking NO or YES. Then please mark the box which best describes how much change there is, if any, from your usual self.

	NO	YES	Much less than usual	Less than usual	No change	More than usual	Much more than usual
1. Tearful							
2. Mentally tense							
3. Able to concentrate							
4. Low spirited							
5. Elated							
6. Helpless							
7. Finding it difficult to show feelings							
8. Alert							
9. Forgetful, muddled							
10. Anxious							
11. Wishing you were alone							
12. Mentally relaxed							
13. Brooding on things							
14. Feeling sorry for yourself							
15. Emotionally numb							
16. Depressed							
17. Over-emotional							
18. Happy							
19. Confident							
20. Changeable in your spirits							
21. Tired							
22. Irritable							
23. Crying without being able to stop							
24. Lively							
25. Over-sensitive							
26. Up and down in mood							
27. Restless							
28. Calm, tranquil							

References

1. Taylor A. (1986) Maternity Services: The consumer's view. *Journal of the Royal College of General Practitioners*. **36**: 157–60.

2. Ball J. (1987) Reactions to motherhood. Cambridge University Press, Cambridge. 53–76.

3. Oakley A and Rajan L. (1990) Obstetric technology and emotional well-being. *Journal of Reproductive and Infant Psychology*. **8**: 45–55.

4. Glover V. (1992) Do biochemical factors play a part in postnatal depression? *Progress in Neuro-Psychopharmacology and Biological Psychiatry*. **16**: 605–15.

5. Parry B. (1992) In: *Recent advances in childbearing and mental health*. Abstracts of the 6th International Conference of the Marcé Society. p. 8.

6. Kendell RE, McGuire RJ, Connor Y, *et al*. (1981) Mood changes in the first three weeks after childbirth. *Journal of Affective Disorders*. **3**: 317–26.

7. Stein G, Marsh A and Morton J. (1981) Mental symptoms, weight change and electrolyte excretion during the first postpartum week. *Journal of Psychosomatic Research*. **25**: 395–408.

8. Robin A. (1962) The psychological changes of normal parturition. *Psychiatric Quarterly*. **36**: 129–50.

9. Stein G. (1980) The pattern of mental changes and body weight change in the first post-partum week. *Journal of Psychosomatic Research*. **24**: 165–71.

10. Kennerley H and Gath D. (1989) Maternity blues: I. Detection and measurement by questionnaire. *British Journal of Psychiatry*. **155**: 356–62.

11. York R. (1990) Pattern of postpartum blues. *Journal of Reproductive and Infant Psychology*. **8**: 67–73.

12. Pitt B. (1968) Atypical depression following childbirth. *British Journal of Psychiatry*. **114**: 1325–35.

13. Knight RG and Thirkettle JA. (1987) The relationship between expectations of pregnancy and birth, and transient depression in the immediate post-partum period. *Journal of Psychosomatic Research*. **31**: 351–7.

14. Hannah P, Adams D, Lee A, *et al.* (1992) Links between early postpartum mood and postnatal depression. *British Journal of Psychiatry*. **160**: 777–80.

15. Thune-Larsen K-B and Moller-Pedersen K. (1988) Childbirth experience and post-partum emotional disturbance. *Journal of Reproductive and Infant Psychology*. **6**: 229–40.

16. Iles S, Gath D and Kennerley H. (1989) Maternity blues: II. Comparison between post-operative and post-natal women. *British Journal of Psychiatry*. **155**: 363–6.

17. Kendell R. Emotional and physical factors in the genesis of puerperal mental disorders. *Journal of Psychosomatic Research*. **29**: 3–11.

18. Davidson JRT. (1972) Post-partum mood change in Jamaican women. *British Journal of Psychiatry*. **121**: 659–63.

19. Condon J and Watson T. (1987) The maternity blues: Exploration of a psychological hypothesis. *Acta Psychiatrica Scandinavica*. **76**: 164–71.

20. Harris B. (1981) Maternity blues in East African clinic attenders. *Archives of General Psychiatry*. **38**: 1293–5.

21. Morsbach G, Sawaragi I, Riddell C, *et al.* (1983) The occurrence of maternity blues in Scottish and Japanese mothers. *Journal of Reproductive and Infant Psychology*. **1**: 29–35.

22. Nott PN, Franklin M, Armitage C, *et al.* (1976) Hormonal changes and mood in the puerperium. *British Journal of Psychiatry*. **128**: 379–83.

23. Feksi A, Harris B, Walker RF, *et al.* (1984) 'Maternity blues' and hormone levels in saliva. *Journal of Affective Disorders*. **6**: 351–55.

24. Okano T and Nomura J. (1990) Endocrine studies of the maternity blues. *Clinical Neuropharmacology*. **13** (Suppl. 2): 532–3.

25. Ehlert U, Patalla U, Kirschbaum C, et al. (1990) Postpartum blues: Salivary cortisol and psychological factors. Journal of Psychosomatic Research. **34**: 319–25.

26. George AJ, Copeland JRM and Wilson KCM. (1980) Prolactin in the maternity blues. British Journal of Pharmacology. **70**: 102–3.

27. Handley SL, Dunn TL, Baker JM, et al. (1977) Mood changes in the puerperium and plasma tryptophan and cortisol concentrations. British Medical Journal. **ii**: 18–20.

28. Harris B. (1980) Prospective trial of L-tryptophan in maternity blues. British Journal of Psychiatry. **137**: 233–5.

29. Hannah P, Adams D, Glover V, et al. (1992) Abnormal platelet 5-hydroxytryptamine uptake and imipramine binding in postnatal dysphoria. Journal of Psychiatric Research. **26**: 69–75.

30. Metz A, Stump K, Cowen P, et al. (1983) Changes in platelet alpha-2-receptor binding post-partum: Possible relation to maternity blues. Lancet. **1**: 495–8.

4   Postnatal Depression

Postnatal depression (PND) is a common condition, occurring in 10–20% of all newly delivered mothers at some stage within the first postnatal year. Far from being the 'happy event' that all women wish for, in these mothers childbirth is often the precipitating factor for a prolonged period of poor mental health, which may have further consequences in terms of marital disharmony and emotional problems in the children.

Is it Postnatal?

Timing

The term 'postnatal' has no implication other than the timing of the illness, and is ill defined, even in this respect. It would be helpful if there were a consensus of opinion about the length of the postnatal period. Some researchers have limited their study to instances occurring in the first six weeks after delivery, some within three months, and some within six months or even one year (Table 4.1)[1-11].

There is some evidence that the physical changes associated with the puerperium, such as weight and disturbances of menstruation, are long lasting, and that women do not achieve their pre-pregnant state until a year after delivery[12].

In addition, large community studies matching obstetric and psychiatric case registers have found a large increase in new cases of psychiatric illness within the first three months post-partum, but also a secondary increase between 10 and 24 months[13]. Taking these physical and psychiatric studies together, it would seem reasonable to include those illnesses with an onset within a year of childbirth under the 'postnatal' umbrella.

Author(s) (year)	Sample size (country)	Postnatal prevalence (%)	Timing
Wolkind et al. (1980)[1]	117 (UK)	10.0 18.0	4 months 14 months
Cox et al. (1982)[2]	105 (Scotland)	13.0	4 months
Cox (1983)[3]	183 (Uganda)	10.0	3 months
Cutrona (1983)[4]	85 (USA)	8.2	8 weeks
Kumar and Robson (1984)[5]	119 (UK)	14.9 11.2 6.5	3 months 6 months 12 months
O'Hara, et al. (1984)[6]	99 (USA)	12.0	9 weeks
Watson, et al. (1984)[7]	128 (UK)	12.0 22.0	6 weeks 12 months
Cooper, et al. (1988)[8]	483 (UK)	8.7 8.8 5.2	3 months 6 months 12 months
Ballard, et al. (1992)[9]	178 (UK)	27.5 25.7	6 weeks 6 months
Kelly and Deakin (1992)[10]	100 (UK)	15.0	2 months
Cox, et al. (1993)[11]	232 (UK)	9.1	6 months

Table 4.1 Recent prevalence studies

Cause or Coincidence?

Few of the studies summarized above (Table 4.1) have included control groups for comparison. We know from sociological studies that there is a high incidence of depression in women in the community in general, and that this is more common where the woman is not in paid work, where there is no confiding relationship, and three or more children under the age of 16 are living at home[14]. Many postnatal women fit into this framework.

We also know that there is a high incidence of psychiatric morbidity in women during pregnancy. Is PND therefore a simple continuation of pre-existing symptoms, or does it differ from other forms of non-psychotic depression in any way except its timing?

A prospective study of 128 women revealed that 29 were 'cases' at some stage during pregnancy or the postnatal year[7]. Of these, 12 had been depressed at some stage during the pregnancy; 17 had a new onset after delivery, but six of the latter showed a pre-existing vulnerability in terms of an episode of psychiatric illness treated by the general practitioner prior to the pregnancy.

One recent study in the USA has used a control group recruited from non-pregnant friends of the pregnant women[6]. The authors found no difference between the two groups in the prevalence rates of depression, but noted that the child-bearing women had higher levels of poor social adjustment and depressive symptoms than their non-child-bearing friends.

Similarly, a controlled study in the UK has shown no difference in point prevalence of depression between postnatal and control subjects at six months, but there was a threefold increase in depressive episodes occurring within five weeks of childbirth[11].

Thus postnatal illnesses tend to be 'clustered' in terms of timing of onset early in the puerperium rather than evenly spread throughout the postnatal year.

Of course, even though the control subjects used in these surveys had not had a baby within the previous 12 months, they are likely to be young women with young children; hence a proportion may be experiencing long-term PND themselves.

Taking all this evidence together suggests that there is a

vulnerability factor, related to previous personality, genetic endowment, or pre-existing psychosocial stress, which, combined with the added stress of pregnancy, delivery and child care, can precipitate PND at some stage within the first postnatal year.

Clearly, the greater the vulnerability, the lower the stress levels required to provoke symptoms. Hence the need to identify women at risk early in the pregnancy so that appropriate intervention can be offered to minimize the inevitable stress of transition to parenthood.

It seems most likely that what we currently call PND is a heterogeneous group of psychiatric illnesses. Some are recurrences or continuations of previous psychiatric disorder, some are a response to stressful life events unrelated to childbirth, some relate to the added stress of child care and responsibility in those ill-prepared for it, and a small proportion occur in women with no predisposing factors, in whom the illness appears to be 'pure' PND.

Is it Depression?

The classical presentation of PND is not very different from the symptoms of depression occurring at other times, although some of the typical features may be confused by the simultaneous physical and environmental changes associated with the puerperal state.

Symptoms to enquire for are:

- persistent low mood
- anxiety and irritability
- sleep disturbance
- lack of energy and enthusiasm
- poor appetite
- inability to cope with daily chores
- poor concentration and memory.

Low Mood

Sad and gloomy mood is usually accompanied by tearfulness, hopelessness or despair, or even a feeling that life is not worth living. Suicidal thoughts do occur, but are generally firmly resisted 'for the sake of the baby', and we know that actual suicide is six times less common in the postnatal year in comparison with women of similar age. Nevertheless, many women will express a wish to 'run away' from their homes and families. Running away can sometimes be a suicidal equivalent in childhood and adolescence, and it may have a similar meaning in PND:

> 'Sometimes I wish I could go somewhere on my own for a week, like a retreat, and just cry and cry and cry and get it all out of my system.'

Unlike other forms of depression, PND is often very variable from day to day. Thus the mother who makes an appointment to see her family doctor or health visitor because she is feeing utterly wretched, may, on the day of the appointment, feel much better, and not wish to admit to her previous despair. It is often more helpful to ask how many days in each week she feels low and miserable, and to offer her open access to the surgery or clinic when these symptoms occur.

Classical depression is characterized by being worse in the morning, and improving as the day goes on. PND seems to reach a peak in late afternoon and early evening, perhaps because at that time the mother is exhausted and the children fractious and ready for bed.

Low mood is usually accompanied by loss of enjoyment in normally happy activities. Women with PND will often avoid social contact, refusing to answer the doorbell or the telephone:

> 'I was grateful that several people befriended me, but was unable to respond because I was so completely absorbed in my misery. A neighbour invited me to her son's birthday party but I was panic-stricken and just couldn't face it.'

Trivial incidents can provoke major outbursts of tearfulness, and there is a powerful identification with the subjects of accidents and natural disasters in the world at large:

'I watched a television programme about nuclear war, and I wept bitterly and deeply, as I could not bear to think of death after giving birth.'

They will wonder at other people who can smile and laugh when the world seems such a gloomy place.

Depression is often accompanied by intense guilt and self-blame. Women feel inadequate and ashamed of feeling the way they do, as if they have failed in the feminine role.

'The most overwhelming feeling was one of total failure. I felt totally inadequate as a mother – me, who'd been a competent teacher, yet now couldn't even cope with one baby. Coupled with all this was the shame I felt – even after I was having medical treatment. I got sick of being told to pull myself together. That's just what you can't do.'

Anxiety and Irritability

This is a common accompaniment to depressed mood. The depressed mother will be over-anxious about minor feeding problems or her baby's health or weight, or may be unable to leave the baby with others. She is unable to tolerate her baby crying. She may worry unduly about financial matters, and be unable to share her feelings with family and friends for fear of over-burdening them, thus increasing her isolation and loneliness:

'I hated my husband going to work. I was afraid that he would be killed at a time when I most needed him.'

Heightened anxiety may give rise to panic attacks, usually when out of the house, but often when alone with the baby. These consist of a feeling of dread, palpitations, difficulty in breathing, trembling and 'butterflies in the stomach'. They are truly alarming if the cause is not understood, and the mother may feel that she is about to die.

Other manifestations of anxiety include feelings that she herself is detached from reality, and simply going through the motions of living, or that the world around her has an 'unreal' quality:

> 'I've had an episode of emptiness – it feels like I cease to exist emotionally for myself – but I am still there for others to react to. In my mind it was as if I was a flat one-dimensional cardboard image of myself.'

The relationship between anxiety and depression in PND is unclear. It may be that depression lowers the threshold for anxiety, or, alternatively, that being constantly anxious and unable to cope leads to a secondary depressive state.

Irritability is rarely experienced towards the baby; it is much more likely to be directed at the partner or the older children. It often worries the mother more than it does her family, and she may experience considerable guilt about her impatience with toddlers. The fear of being a 'child batterer' is ever present in the minds of these mothers and may even reach the level of obsessional ruminations.

Sleep Disturbance

This is difficult to assess in a mother who may be breast-feeding throughout the night.

The characteristic sleep disturbance of depression is early morning waking, at 2 or 3am, and being unable to sleep again. These mothers are more likely to experience difficulty in getting off to sleep, being unable to 'unwind' from the stress of the day, and, when woken by the baby, will find it difficult to get back to sleep again. Even if the baby sleeps through the night, the mother will often wake several times, commonly getting into a deep stage of sleep in the early morning, and finding it difficult to rouse herself to face the day:

> 'A bad night – very restless. I had lots of very vivid dreams again, and this last hour all I can think of is the nature of the deaths of people I have known.'

Alternatively, she may feel that she wants to sleep all day, and that no amount of sleep helps her to feel refreshed. This is a 'hibernation' reaction, both a physical slowing up, and an unconscious avoidance of the unpleasant feelings associated with the day:

'When I had weaned the baby at eight months, I began
to realize that I no longer felt well. I had feelings of
inadequacy, I cried for no reason, I was bad-tempered,
I couldn't seem to find the energy for the tasks I had
done competently for several months. Getting up in the
morning was the worst. I just wanted to crawl back
under the bedclothes.'

A mother will often present to the family doctor with sleep
problems, sometimes being treated with tranquillizers such as
diazepam. These only compound the depression, the early
morning sluggishness, and the feeling of being 'out of control'.

Lack of Energy and Enthusiasm

Many mothers report a strange quality to their lack of energy.
They may say that they are aware that the baby needs feeding,
or that domestic chores are piling up, and, although they mentally will themselves to do the tasks, their limbs seem reluctant
to obey. One woman described the feeling 'as if her feet were
stuck in treacle'.

In other forms of depression, mental and physical retardation
seem to change in parallel, but in PND, the physical slowing
seems out of proportion. Perhaps this is why so many women
interpret their feelings in physical terms:

'It wasn't until about nine months after the birth that
I began to notice that I wasn't well at all. I had dreadful
dizzy spells and nausea. I thought I might have cancer,
an allergy, or failing kidneys. I had tests for everything
we could think of, but all seemed to be negative. My
doctor put me on Valium. He said I was naturally
depressed and anxious, and that this was common to
women with their first baby.'

Poor Appetite

This again is difficult to gauge in a new mother who finds that
child care takes up most of the day. Many say that they do not
find time for proper meals, but constantly nibble for comfort on
biscuits and junk food. They then put on weight, feeling fat and
unattractive just when they were hoping to get back to their pre-
pregnant figure.

Some women find it difficult to feed the family, as if, once they have fed the demanding baby, they have nothing good left to give. Others will cook for the family, but are unable to sit down and enjoy a meal themselves, perhaps feeling guilty about even taking the time to eat:

> 'I never seemed to have time to eat or to relax. I began to resent the baby because she never let me have any time to myself. It could take me a day or more just to read a newspaper.'

Inability to Cope

Depression is accompanied by an overwhelming feeling of being unable to cope with day to day activities. This, in a woman who has been active, energetic and capable in her previous working life, is most damaging to her self-esteem. Indecision is a common accompaniment to depression, and these women find great difficulty in even deciding what to wear each day, as well as more important decisions about feeding the baby or establishing a routine for housework.

Far from her imagined image of contented baby sleeping, tidy house, and dinner in the oven, her partner may return from work to find a dishevelled, tearful wife, a crying baby, a chaotic house, and no meal ready. Her constant comparison of the reality with her imagined scenario, and with her fantasy of other mothers coping happily and well, makes her feel a failure as a woman, a wife, and a mother. The guilt is almost unbearable:

> 'People who came round or rang were only interested in the baby, not in me. I felt awful, and just wished that I could get her adopted, or that someone would take her away and not bring her back.'

> 'During the mornings, when I had to be alone at home, I was deeply afraid, felt absolutely devoid of confidence, and very tense. I felt some mornings that I would go crazy. My head felt like it would burst. My body felt as if it wanted to keep moving, so I rocked and rocked in my rocking chair.'

Poor Concentration and Memory

One elderly midwife was in the habit of telling new mothers that they would 'lose a quarter of their brain after each baby'. Although patent nonsense, this is actually how some women feel. They forget what they need at the shops, forget what they went upstairs for, and forget medical appointments. They are unable to concentrate on reading, constantly flicking back pages to remind themselves, and television is just so much 'moving wallpaper'. They find themselves at a loss in conversation, losing the thread, and feeling stupid. The contrast between this and their previous competence at work is devastating to confidence and self-esteem:

> 'I understand that it takes two years to recover from having a baby. It may be true. I still feel a bit vague, and sometimes have slight lapses of memory.'

> 'In retrospect, I can see that I experienced mental confusion. The greatest concentration and willpower were required for even the simplest jobs.'

Loss of Libido

This is a normal occurrence during the postpartum year, and may even be the remnant of a primitive instinct towards suitable spacing of pregnancies. Perineal discomfort and sheer physical exhaustion are also contributory. However, loss of libido is a common symptom of depression, often the first one to appear and the last to remit. It contributes to the mother's guilt about being an inadequate wife, and, if the partner is impatient or intolerant, may lead to further friction and loss of support from him.

Why is the Diagnosis Missed?

PND often seems to be overlooked or inadequately treated, and there are a variety of reasons why this should be so.

Failure of the Mother to Recognize the Syndrome

Many women struggle through the first year with their new baby with a powerful feeling that all is not well, but being unable to identify what is wrong. They may only recognize the problem in retrospect, when they suddenly again find increased energy and pleasure in normal activities, and are able to respond to their babies more positively. They then realize that they have experienced an illness, and are not, as they may have thought, 'simply not cut out for motherhood'.

The symptoms may also be missed because they usually have a gradual onset and, in the early stages, may be confused with normal tiredness and exhaustion created by broken nights and increased physical activity.

In addition, the condition is often fluctuant from day to day, and is therefore often attributed to immediate and practical problems rather than underlying depression:

> 'Thank goodness I didn't suffer as badly as some, although I did have medical treatment in the form of tablets for six months. Even then it took 18 months before I felt 'normal' again. I think the point I would like to make is that I didn't even realize I had PND, and neither did my husband or family. It took an observant health visitor to literally make an appointment for me at the doctor's.'

Refusal of the Mother to Identify the Syndrome

Many women recognize the symptoms in themselves, and are bitterly ashamed of feeling the way they do. They perceive other mothers to be happy and coping well, and feel that only they themselves are failing to enjoy motherhood. They blame themselves for being 'incompetent' or 'inadequate', and fear the consequences if they admit to their real feelings. Perhaps they will be told to 'pull themselves together', or criticized; worse still, they may believe that the baby will be taken into care.

When someone is feeling low in mood, particularly if this is a feeling foreign to them, it is a natural reaction to wish to find a reason. In most women's lives there is something giving rise to sadness or disappointment. This then is used as 'a peg to hang it on' and the supposed reason for the depression is overvalued. Only when they begin to improve can this be seen as a result, rather than the cause, of the illness.

Failure of Primary Carers to Recognize the Syndrome

These women often attempt to get some help by reporting physical symptoms, either in themselves or their babies, feeling that these are more acceptable to the family doctor. This is self-defeating as they will be seen as hypochondriacal and unnecessary attenders at the surgery, and therefore even less likely to get the help they need. The classical presentation is the mother who has attended the surgery on many occasions for trivial complaints. On one of these visits, she may be reluctant to leave, or may burst into tears at the end of the consultation. In the middle of a busy surgery, the family doctor may not be able to give her the time she needs to say how she feels.

A typical mother reports seven weeks after the delivery:

'I still felt constantly tired and even after sleeping I felt physically drained. During the day my limbs felt limp and shaky and I often had dizzy spells. My GP tested me for diabetes and thyroid imbalance, but these all proved to be negative. He then admitted that I was a puzzle to him, but said that it would probably pass and I should just plod on.'

This woman eventually took a serious overdose, and spent a week in a psychiatric hospital followed by out-patient treatment. She made a full recovery when her baby was a year old.

Health visitors are traditionally child orientated and are advice-givers. During her home visits, the mother may make special efforts to seem happy and competent. It takes a great deal of perception and previous knowledge of the mother to recognize the falsity of the image presented, and it needs time and attention to the mother's needs to persuade her to reveal how she really feels. One mother said:

'My depression following my first pregnancy escalated due to the fact that nobody was there to see the warning signs.'

Reluctance of Primary Carers to Recognize the Syndrome

The midwife and health visitor will probably not have been trained in mental health problems, and may feel at a loss to know how to help. Their own feelings of ignorance and helplessness may even lead them to avoid the depressed mother, compounding the problem still further.

Even if the family doctor recognizes that the mother is severely distressed, they may have had little training or experience in the treatment of PND, may be concerned about giving medication if the mother is breast-feeding, or have little knowledge of local support groups or counselling facilities. The general practitioner will recognize that the illness is relatively mild, and probably transient. The doctor may therefore be reluctant to refer the mother to a psychiatrist, especially as there is rarely a local consultant with a particular interest in postnatal problems.

Failure of Psychiatric Services to Recognize the Syndrome

Only 19% of district psychiatric services have specialized in-patient facilities for mother and baby admissions, and only 40% have a consultant with a particular interest in postnatal disorders[15]. Even these consultants may be primarily concerned with major psychiatric illness, such as psychoses and personality disorders, and may find the milder, neurotic illnesses occurring in the postnatal year trivial by comparison. There are exceedingly few specialists who devote their whole time to perinatal psychiatric problems.

These depressed mothers may not then get the attention they deserve, either from primary or secondary care systems. This is a tragedy in terms of the prolonged morbidity that can follow, with consequent implications for effects on the child[16,17] and the integrity of the family[18].

Making the Diagnosis

The most important factor is for health professionals to be aware of and sensitive to, the feelings of newly delivered mothers. No woman will confide in a health visitor or family doctor who is impatient, in a hurry, or only interested in the baby. Good listening skills are essential, and non-verbal communication is equally important. Open ended questions will elicit useful information, and the professional's response should be empathic and non-directive.

Aspects of care which women have found helpful include:

- listening

- sounding as if he/she cared

- not being judgmental

- being willing to give time

- being able to detect feelings not expressed in words

- accepting good and bad feelings

- being encouraging, giving praise for effort

- showing confidence.

Many attempts have been made to find a suitable screening questionnaire for PND. Most of the existing instruments were developed to rate degrees of depression, rather than to distinguish between normality and psychiatric illness. Many were found to be unsatisfactory because of the inclusion of somatic symptoms which may relate to the postnatal state rather than to PND. Some were unacceptable in terms of length, both to postnatal women and primary care workers, and some, such as the Beck Depression Inventory, which is geared to the more severe end of the spectrum, were not sensitive enough.

The Edinburgh Postnatal Depression Scale (EPDS; Appendix 4.1)[19] was developed to counteract these difficulties. Over a considerable length of time it has been found to be acceptable to clients and professionals alike, to be quick to complete and to score, and, most importantly, to have both a high sensitivity (95%) and specificity (93%); that is, it correctly identifies the majority of mothers with PND, and does not include a large number of 'false positives'. Another advantage is that, because it is a self-rating scale, it does not depend on the judgement or training of the observer.

There are some important points to be borne in mind when using the EPDS.

* It was developed as a screening instrument, not a diagnostic tool. Using it therefore simply to 'confirm' depression where it is already suspected, is inappropriate.

* A single high score on the EPDS may simply reflect transient problems. It is therefore recommended that high scorers should repeat the test after one or two weeks, and the results only be considered significant if both scores are high.

* Women may not answer the questionnaire truthfully if they are ashamed of their feelings, or afraid that the children may be removed from them.

* If it is used in an impersonal and routine way, women may feel that there is no true concern about them as individuals, and look upon it simply as an authoritarian 'checking-up' on them as mothers.

* Health carers may see the use of a questionnaire as a substitute, rather than a facilitator for empathic listening and observation.

* Labelling the mother as having a psychiatric illness carries a stigma, and 'medicalizes' the condition. It may also block practical and cognitive intervention which could prevent a downward spiralling of the depression.

* The anxiety of health professionals is raised by the positive answers to the self-harm question.

* There is no point in screening for a condition if no help is available. A suitable hierarchy of intervention strategies should be in place before screening begins.

Course and Outcome of PND

Surprisingly, little research has been carried out into the natural history of the illness. Anecdotal reports from women who have suffered PND indicate that, untreated, the illness may persist for at least one or two years. There are also suggestions that, on recovery, women may suffer from 'mini relapses' at each premenstrual period, thus supporting the hormonal theories of aetiology.

In prospective studies, over 50% of depressed mothers have been shown to have an illness lasting three months or more, and 30% have illnesses lasting six months or more[7]; 40–50% of mothers diagnosed as depressed at six weeks postpartum were still depressed at six months[5,7].

One follow-up study[20] showed that 43% of depressed mothers had made little recovery by one year postpartum, and another that 63% of women for whom the postpartum disorder was their first psychiatric illness were still significantly impaired at 14 months[1].

An audit of mothers at high risk for the development of PND up to five years postpartum showed that approximately one-third still had scores above the cut-off point for depression on the EPDS[21]. There was no correlation of the scores with time from delivery, suggesting that these women suffered from a chronic depressive disorder.

Another review of mothers four years after the birth of a child[5] showed that new cases of depression occurring at any time during pregnancy or the first postnatal year correlated with an increased incidence of psychiatric consultations up to three years later. The authors conclude that '... for some women, childbearing heralds the start of prolonged emotional difficulties'. This rather gloomy prognosis was applied to women in a prospective study who were not in treatment. It is to be hoped that, with improved levels of identification and treatment both in primary and psychiatric care, the prospects are now brighter for such women.

Recurrence Rate

In comparison with puerperal psychosis, where the recurrence rate has been extensively researched, there is little published information about the recurrence of PND after subsequent pregnancies. One author quotes 68% in an untreated sample[22], and another[23] puts it as high as 75%. A third also suggests that it may recur in a more severe and prolonged form with subsequent episodes[24].

Leverton and Elliott[25] identified a 'high risk' group of pregnant women on the basis of a variety of factors including previous PND. Half the sample were offered 'preparation for parenthood' classes, together with individual support and training in stress management. The prevalence of PND in those offered the intervention was 19%, compared with 40% in the remainder.

A more recent audit of women with previous postnatal depression, who were identified antenatally and offered preventative intervention, showed that the recurrence rate of PND was 50%, which was similar to that of women with previous non-puerperal psychiatric illness[21].

Appendix 4.1

The Edinburgh Postnatal Depression Scale

Name: Date:
Address: Age:
                                   Date of delivery:

As you have recently had a baby, we would like to know how you are feeling now. Please UNDERLINE the answer that comes closest to how you have felt IN THE PAST WEEK.

Here is an example, already completed.

I have felt happy:
  Yes, all the time
  <u>Yes, most of the time</u>
  No, not very often
  No, not at all

This would mean: 'I have felt happy most of the time' during the past week.
Please complete the other questions in the same way.

IN THE PAST 7 DAYS

1   I have been able to laugh and see the funny side of things
    As much as I always could
    Not quite so much now
    Definitely not so much now
    Not at all

2   I have looked forward with enjoyment to things
      As much as I ever did
      Rather less than I used to
      Definitely less than I used to
      Hardly at all

3*   I have blamed myself unnecessarily when things went wrong
      Yes, most of the time
      Yes, some of the time
      Not very often
      No, never

4   I have been anxious and worried for no good reason
      No, not at all
      Hardly ever
      Yes, sometimes
      Yes, very often

5*   I have felt scared or panicky for no very good reason
      Yes, quite a lot
      Yes, sometimes
      No, not much
      No, not all

6*   Things have been getting on top of me
      Yes, most of the time I haven't been able to cope at all
      Yes, sometimes I haven't been coping as well as usual
      No, most of the time I have coped quite well
      No, I have been coping as well as ever

7*   I have been so unhappy that I have had difficulty sleeping
      Yes, most of the time
      Yes, sometimes
      Not very often
      No, not at all

8*   I have felt sad or miserable
      Yes, most of the time
      Yes, quite often
      Not very often
      No, not at all

9*　I have been so unhappy that I have been crying
　　Yes, most of the time
　　Yes, quite often
　　Only occasionally
　　No, never

10*　The thought of harming myself has occurred to me
　　Yes, quite often
　　Sometimes
　　Hardly ever
　　Never

Scoring:
　Items are scored 0, 1, 2, or 3.
　Questions marked * are reverse scored: 3, 2, 1 or 0.
　Scores of 12 or above distinguish borderline and probable cases from non-cases.

References

1. Wolkind S, Zajicek E and Ghodsian M. (1980) Continuities in maternal depression. *International Journal of Family Psychiatry.* 1: 167–82.

2. Cox JL, Connor Y and Kendell RE. (1982) Prospective study of the psychiatric disorders of childbirth. *British Journal of Psychiatry.* 140: 111-7.

3. Cox JL. (1983) Postnatal depression: A comparison of African and Scottish women. *Social Psychiatry.* 18: 25–8.

4. Cutrona CE. (1983) Causal attributions and postnatal depression. *Journal of Abnormal Psychiatry.* 92: 161–72.

5. Kumar R and Robson KM. (1984) A prospective study of emotional disorders in childbearing women. *British Journal of Psychiatry.* 144: 35–47.

6. O'Hara MW, Neunaber DJ and Zekoski EM. (1984) A prospective study of postpartum depression: Prevalence, course and predictive factors. *Journal of Abnormal Psychology.* 93: 158–71.

7. Watson JP, Elliott SA, Rugg AJ, *et al.* (1984) Psychiatric disorder in pregnancy and the first postnatal year. *British Journal of Psychiatry.* 144: 453–62.

8. Cooper PJ, Campbell EA, Day A, *et al.* (1988) Non-psychotic psychiatric disorder after childbirth. *British Journal of Psychiatry.* 152: 799–806.

9. Ballard C, Davis R and Cullen PC, *et al.* (1992) Postnatal depression in mothers and fathers. In: *Recent advances in childbearing and mental health.* Abstracts of the 6th International Conference of the Marcé Society. *British Journal of Psychiatry.* 164: 782–8.

10. Kelly A and Deakin JFW. (1992) Psychosocial and biological predictors of early postnatal depression. In: *Recent advances in childbearing and mental health.* Abstracts of the 6th International Conference of the Marcé Society. 23.

11. Cox JL, Murray D and Chapman G. (1993) A controlled study of the onset, duration and prevalence of postnatal depression. *British Journal of Psychiatry.* **163**: 27–31.

12. Jacobson L, Kaij L and Nilsson A. (1967) The course and outcome of the postpartum period from a gynaecological and general somatic standpoint. *Acta Obstetrica et Gynecologica Scandinavica.* **46**: 183–203.

13. Kendell RE, Wainwright S, Hailey A, *et al.* (1976) The influence of childbirth on psychiatric morbidity. *Psychological Medicine.* **6**: 297–302.

14. Brown GW and Harris T. (1978) *The social origins of depression: A study of psychiatric disorders in women.* Free Press, New York.

15. Prettyman RJ and Friedman T. (1991) Care of women with puerperal psychiatric disorders in England and Wales. *British Medical Journal.* **302**: 1245–6.

16. Cogill SA, Caplan H, Alexandra H, *et al.* (1986) Impact of maternal postnatal depression on the cognitive development of the young child. *British Medical Journal.* **292**: 1165–7.

17. Caplan H, Cogill SR, Alexandra H, *et al.* (1989) Maternal depression and the emotional development of the child. *British Journal of Psychiatry.* **154**: 818–22.

18. Rutter M and Quinton D. (1984) Parental psychiatric disorder: Effects on children. *Psychological Medicine.* **14**: 853–80.

19. Cox JL, Holden J and Sagovsky R. (1987) Detection of postnatal depression: Development of the 10-item Edinburgh Postnatal Depression Scale. *British Journal of Psychiatry.* **150**: 782–6.

20. Pitt B. (1968) Atypical depression following childbirth. *British Journal of Psychiatry.* **114**: 1325–35.

21. Quinton C and Riley DM. (1993) Does psychiatric consultation in pregnancy prevent postnatal depression? *Auditorium.* **2**: 58–62.

22. Dalton K. (1985) Progesterone prophylaxis used successfully in postnatal depression. *Practitioner.* **229**: 507–8.

23. Garvey MJ, Tuason VB, Lumry AE, *et al.* (1983) Occurrence of depression in the postpartum state. *Journal of Affective Disorders.* **5**: 97–101.

24. Kaij L, Jacobson L and Nilsson A. (1967) Postpartum mental disorder in an unselected sample: The influence of parity. *Journal of Psychosomatic Research*; **10**: 317–25.

25. Leverton TJ and Elliott SA. (1989) Transition to parenthood groups: A preventative intervention for postnatal depression. In: van Hall EV and Everaerd W, editors. *The free woman: Women's health in the 1990s*. Parthenon Press, Carnforth, Lancs, 479–86.

5 What Causes Postnatal Depression?

Many research studies have attempted to unravel the complicated constellation of events leading to PND. Until recently it was a poorly defined condition, and diagnostic criteria have varied from study to study. Researchers have often pursued individual facets of the aetiology, depending on their own interests, rather than looking at the situation as a whole.

The often conflicting views on causation almost certainly reflect the fact that it is a heterogenous group of disorders, probably multifactorial in origin. The contributory causes can be classified under the following headings:

- socio-demographic: age, social class, life events, partner support etc.

- obstetric/gynaecological: eg previous or recent obstetric or gynaecological events

- personality factors: neuroticism, overdependency, anxious or depressive personality

- psychiatric factors: previous psychiatric illness in the mother or in her family; previous premenstrual syndrome and 'blues'

- biological factors: changes in hormones and neurotransmitters related to pregnancy and after

- factors related to the infant: prematurity, ill health, fractious baby.

Socio-demographic Factors

Age

Several studies have found a higher incidence in older mothers (ie those over 30 years of age)[1,2], and also in younger mothers[3] [-7]. This is understandable in terms of the older mothers having a greater adjustment to make, and the younger ones possibly being more socially disadvantaged. One survey revealed a higher incidence in 'young multiparae', ie those under the age of 31 with three or more children[8].

Social Class

There is overwhelming evidence that PND is not necessarily related to social class. It appears to be just as common in women in social classes 1 and 2 as in working-class mothers[5,8,9,10,11]. Since most of the studies are prospective, aimed at detecting psychiatric symptoms in community samples, we cannot assume that the higher social class mothers are simply more vocal about their distress. The equality of spread across social class barriers is therefore real, and in sharp contrast to the findings in other community surveys, that depression is more common in social classes 4 and 5.

The clue to this enigma may lie in the obvious buffering effect of social support systems. It may be that middle class women are more likely to move away from the parental neighbourhood for educational and career reasons, and are therefore less likely to have close confiding relationships with family, friends and neighbours. They may also have higher expectations of childbirth and motherhood, and be less likely, for financial reasons, to return to work within the first postnatal year. There is evidence from sociological studies that paid part-time work outside the home is protective against depression[12].

All mothers previously working outside the home are likely to experience the loss of adult company and the time and money for leisure pursuits, but there is also evidence that the woman who has had a career in which she was successful and happy is more likely to experience loss of status, income and intellectual stimulation on becoming a mother. Western society seems to expect women to adapt to an isolated existence within their own homes, and to give up their previous freedom without regret or sadness. Other cultures seem to have a more realistic view, arranging for the mother to be 'nurtured' herself for several weeks after childbirth; even in less industrialized western societies there is more often a large extended family who share in the later child rearing.

Marital Status

This seems to have little importance, perhaps because of the large preponderance of married subjects in most of the studies, and because it is increasingly acceptable in society to be a single mother. Not all single mothers are unsupported; many are in a long-term secure relationship, and it is the quality rather than the legality of the relationship that is important.

Disharmony Within the Relationship

Do women become depressed because of relationship difficulties, or is their account of the relationship distorted unfavourably because they are depressed? Until we have a truly prospective study looking at these factors before the beginning of pregnancy, we shall not be sure. Most of the studies have investigated women from early pregnancy onwards.

We know that pregnancy depression can be related to post-natal symptoms, so it may be that these women were already depressed and therefore viewing partner support in a poor light well before the delivery. We also know that, in a proportion of women, pregnancy is embarked upon to 'mend' a failing relationship, or to provide a love object for the woman who feels unloved. Disappointment with the partner when these ends are not achieved may contribute to PND.

More substantial evidence is supplied by studies which noted an increase in psychiatric symptoms in the partners of depressed women, suggesting that women with partners unable to give support because of their own emotional problems were more likely to develop PND[13,14].

It is a sad fact that, just at the time women have children, their partners are often beginning to establish themselves in a career, and to move up the promotion ladder. They may also be anxious about the loss of income associated with the pregnant woman giving up work. If the father interprets his role mainly as a material provider for the new family, he is likely to work extra hard for longer hours, and is therefore even less available to offer emotional and practical support at precisely the time that his partner needs it.

Life Events and Social Support

Women embarking on pregnancy clearly need a secure background in terms not only of relationships, but also practical issues such as housing and finance. Their pleasure at having the baby will be impaired by knowing that they have only a single room in which to bring up the child, or that they will be financially constrained during its infancy. One large study in three countries showed that housing and financial stress were both significantly related to PND at four months[1].

Some of the conflicting evidence about social disadvantage comes from the fact that surveys have been carried out in very different socio-economic groups. However, even in middle-class populations, where actual deprivation is uncommon, impending childbirth often necessitates a move to a larger house, or an extension to the existing one. Both of these events can be profoundly unsettling in the context of adjustment to a new baby.

In terms of other life events, there is evidence that women bereaved during pregnancy 'postpone' their grief reaction until after the delivery, and that the constellation of birth and death within a short time-scale can be difficult to negotiate[15].

Close Confiding Relationships

Sociological surveys have revealed a higher rate of depression in women with no-one in whom they can confide. In the absence of a suitably close relationship with a partner, a female friend or relative could assume this role.

Women who are socially mobile because of their own or their partner's work may not have been able to make local friends, and those who have been working during pregnancy may only have a circle of friends who are childless and career orientated.

To a large extent, this can be rectified by attending antenatal classes, where contact will be made with other mothers due to have their babies at about the same time, or by attending mother and toddler groups arranged by health visitors or social workers. However, if these mothers are already depressed during the pregnancy, they may have difficulty in making new relationships. One to one befriending, such as that provided by the National Childbirth Trust or the Association for Postnatal Illness, may therefore be more appropriate.

'Social support' is a rather vague term, and many of the studies quoted do not specify the measures used. One recent study[16] developed a questionnaire to elucidate the type of support which women can feel comfortable with. The statements with which women are invited to identify include:

- Even if my parents lived far away I know that if I were in need I would be able to depend on them

- If I am upset or confused I know there is always someone I can turn to

- There is always someone with whom I can share my happiness and excitement

- I believe in times of difficulty my neighbours would help me.

This study compared women in Britain and in Greece, and found that social support and life events were the major predictors of postpartum depressed mood in both cultures.

Relationship With Own Mother

Childbirth is often accompanied by a strong identification with, and dependence on, the woman's own mother. Where she is either geographically or emotionally distant, problems are more likely to occur. Equally damaging is the critical or over-intrusive mother, who undermines her confidence (*see* Case Study 5.1).

The woman's own experience of mothering may also be relevant. A woman whose own mother may have been undemonstrative, inconsistent, or preoccupied with work or the care of a large family, will have no satisfactory role model when she becomes a mother herself. She also has the dilemma of wanting to be the 'perfect' mother in contrast to her own experience, yet perhaps experiencing some envy of her own child for having what she herself missed.

Problems in her own childhood which may have been 'buried' during her adult life may be reactivated by her identification with her own baby, resulting in a resurgence of anger at her own parents, just at a time when she most needs support from them. This kind of reaction is particularly common in women who have experienced sexual abuse in childhood. Another suggested explanation is that women with greater childhood problems may have greater current social difficulties.

Research Findings

The often contradictory findings from research studies are summarized in Table 5.1 The apparent inconsistencies shown here reflect differences in the criteria used to define PND, together with generally small sample size and low incidence rate. Nevertheless, there is a general consensus that those factors, such as adverse life events, poor socio-economic status and lack of support from the partner, family and friends, are confirmed in these studies overleaf.

Obstetric or Gynaecological Factors Associated with PND

Menstrual Problems

Dysmenorrhoea and irregular menstruation have been cited as predisposing factors for PND[32]. The psychoanalytical interpretation of this connection has been in terms of 'rejection of the feminine role'. An equally valid interpretation is that both are more frequent in women with high neuroticism scores on personality questionnaires, and it may be that psychological vulnerability predisposes to both. Alternatively, dysmenorrhoea may be connected with particularly painful labour which may also be relevant to postnatal distress.

Risk factor	Studies finding increased risk		Studies finding no increased risk	
Young mothers	Hayworth	1980[3]	Pitt	1968[30]
	Paykel	1980[4]	Martin	1977[19]
	Feggetter	1981[5]		
	Handley	1980[6]		
	Zajicek	1978[7]		
Older mothers	Dennerstein	1989[1]		
	Kumar	1984[2]		
Socio-economic status	Ballard	1992[9]	Haysworth	1980[3]
	Feggetter	1981[5]	Watson	1984[23]
	Playfair	1981[10]	Martin	1989[27]
	Campbell	1991[11]	Green	1990[31]
Marital status	Feggetter	1981[5]	Martin	1989[27]
	Pfost	1990[17]	Watson	1984[23]
	O'Hara	1984[18]	Hayworth	1980[3]
Marital disharmony	Martin	1977[19]	Anzalone	1977[32]
	Ballinger	1982[20]	Blair	1970[33]
	Paykel	1980[4]		
	Feggetter	1981[5]		
	Cutrona	1982[21]		
	Cox	1982[22]		
	Kumar	1984[2]		
	Watson	1984[23]		
	O'Hara	1986[24]		
	Nott	1982[25]		
Poor social support	Paykel	1980[4]	Hopkins	1987[34]
	Cutrona	1982[21]		
	Feggetter	1981[5]		
	O'Hara	1986[24]		
	Thorpe	1992[16]		
Lack of confiding relationship	Martin	1989[27]		
	Paykel	1980[4]		
	Nott	1982[25]		
Poor relationship with own parents	Pound	1985[26]	Paykel	1980[4]
	Nott	1982[25]		
	Kumar	1984[2]		
Housing problems	Paykel	1980[4]	Pitt	1968[30]
	Martin	1989[27]		

Risk factor	Studies finding increased risk		Studies finding no increased risk	
Low income	Cooper	1988[28]	Murray	1992[35]
Low education level	Campbell	1991[11]	Robinson	1989[36]
	O'Hara	1984[18]		
Stressful life events	Paykel	1980[4]	Hopkins	1987[34]
	Cutrona	1983[29]	Kumar	1984[2]
	Playfair	1981[10]		
	O'Hara	1984[18]		
	Dennerstein	1989[1]		
Undesirable life events since birth	Cooper	1988[28]		

Table 5.1 Socio-demographic factors associated with an increased risk of postnatal depression

Previous Infertility

Unsuccessful attempts to become pregnant over a period of time may lead to an overvaluing of pregnancy and childbirth, and a consequent disappointment with the reality. There is even at times a subtle switch from 'wanting a baby' to 'wanting to be pregnant' during the infertile period, as if women come to want affirmation of their own normality and femininity by becoming pregnant, rather than the reality of a child and the subsequent upheaval in their life-style.

Previous Termination, Miscarriage or Neonatal Loss

One investigation related the number of previous pregnancies of under 28 weeks' duration to PND at three months postpartum, but no distinction was made between termination of pregnancy and miscarriage[10]. Another found previous termination to be relevant to depression in pregnancy, but not postpartum[2].

Clinical evidence suggests that women who have terminations before they have children may resolve their feelings adequately at the time. However, when they have a baby later, the reality of the previous termination becomes painful. It can no longer be viewed as a simple evacuation of the uterus, but as the destruction of a 'real baby', together with a resurgence of guilt (*see* Case Study 5.2).

In addition, however the previous pregnancy was lost, the present child is, in some sense, not the first, and there is inevitable speculation about what the 'other' would have been like. More perfect perhaps, since fantasy cannot be challenged, and the current reality compares unfavourably with the absent ideal.

Previous still birth, particularly if unexplained, may give rise to severe anxiety in late pregnancy, and the latter can also correlate with PND. True ambivalence can occur when a woman is rejoicing over a safe delivery and a healthy baby, yet still mourning the previous loss. This has been termed 'shadow grief'.

Previous neonatal death, especially a cot death, can give rise to severe postpartum anxiety about a recurrence, and a resurgence of grief for the lost child[15,37]. There is anecdotal evidence for PND occurring in these women after a subsequent delivery.

Unplanned or Unwanted Pregnancy

Several studies have postulated a connection between PND and unplanned pregnancy, and seem to have had no difficulty in assigning women to one or other group[1,20,38,39]. Other experience has shown that a large proportion of women can give no definitive answer to the question as to whether the pregnancy was planned or not.

Perhaps more relevant is the question of whether the pregnancy was welcome or not. Certainly one research study has related PND to having considered termination in early pregnancy[2].

One connection between the two factors may be the adverse social environment leading both to ambivalence about the pregnancy and to later PND.

Parity

Most studies have found no correlation between PND and parity, and, in those that have, the evidence is equally balanced between finding increased rates of depression in primiparae or in multiparae. However, one has found higher rates in young women having their third or subsequent child[8], and this fits in well with sociological surveys relating the stress of having young children living at home to depression in women[12].

Difficulties in Pregnancy

There is a great deal of published work relating anxiety and depression scores in early pregnancy to postpartum psychiatric illness, but little in terms of the effect of physical complications of pregnancy. One American study found that the most powerful predictors of PND were marital status, antepartum depression and 'difficulty' in pregnancy[17]. The latter was assessed by self-report, and the difficulties were not categorized. One of the pioneering studies in the UK found a significant negative correlation between nausea and vomiting in pregnancy and PND[40]. Pregnancy induced hypertension and anaemia have not been found to be relevant.

Difficulties in Labour

Somewhat surprisingly, the overwhelming consensus of research shows that dissatisfaction with the actuality or the mother's perception of childbirth have little to do with late onset postnatal depression[31,41]. These issues may be related to mood in the early puerperium, but not at a later date.

However, one investigation showed that delivery problems were not related to subsequent postnatal depression in women who were previously psychiatrically well, but, in women with a previous psychiatric history, a complicated delivery increased the risk[42].

There is some evidence that the emotional consequences of caesarian section are less if the operation is carried out under epidural anaesthesia. There may also be a difference in the woman's perception of the operation if it is a planned section rather than an emergency procedure[43,44].

It is somewhat surprising also, that women appear to tolerate better, and recover more quickly from, caesarian section than from hysterectomy, which is broadly similar in terms of physical scarring and postoperative pain. Few surgeons would expect post-hysterectomy patients to leave hospital after five days, and resume normal home activities, much less the extra physical demands of lifting, carrying and feeding a new baby. Perhaps the answer lies in the emotional implications of each operation: a gain for caesarian section, and a loss for hysterectomy.

Perhaps, too, we should make more help available to women having had a section, or allow a longer hospital stay if there is inadequate help in the home.

Breast-feeding

One study has shown that unsupplemented breast feeding until three months postpartum is related to depressed mood[45]. This may be due to the nutritional drain on the mother, but is more likely to be as a result of more frequent feeds, especially at night, and the fact that the mother is solely responsible for feeding, with no possibility of help from others. These women may also experience a longer period of suppression of ovarian activity.

Other mothers report sadness at the failure of breast-feeding, and one study associates bottle-feeding with a higher rate of depression at six weeks postpartum[46].

Anecdotally, there is a small group of mothers whose depression begins as breast-feeding ceases, but, since both events may occur during the first postpartum year, the association is likely to be coincidental.

Research Findings

Studies concerning the association between obstetric and gynaecological factors and the risk of PND are listed in Table 5.2.

Personality and Psychiatric Factors Associated with PND

Personality Characteristics

There are various psychological questionnaires designed to elicit aspects of personality. Two of these, the Maudsley Personality Inventory and the Eysenck Personality Questionnaire, have been used in attempts to define individual vulnerability to

Risk factor	Studies finding increased risk		Studies finding no increased risk	
Menstrual problems	Playfair	1981[10]		
	Pitt	1968[30]		
Previous infertility	Kumar	1984[2]		
Previous termination of	Playfair	1981[10]	Paykel	1980[4]
pregnancy or miscarriage	Kumar	1984[2]	Watson	1984[23]
Previous neonatal loss	Clarke	1979[15]		
Unplanned or unwanted	Martin	1977[19]		
pregnancy	Braverman	1978[39]		
	Dennerstein	1989[1]		
	Nilsson	1967[38]		
Considered termination of pregnancy	Kumar	1984[2]		
Parity				
High	Playfair	1981[10]	Paykel	1980[4]
Low	Bridge	1985[47]	Hayworth	1980[3]
			Cox	1982[22]
			Watson	1984[23]
Difficult pregnancy	Pfost	1990[17]		
Fear of childbirth	Areskog	1984[48]		
	Dennerstein	1989[1]		
Obstetric complications	Oakley	1980[42]	Paykel	1980[4]
	Dean	1981[49]	Cox	1982[22]
	Ballinger	1982[20]	Gennaro	1988[50]
	Cutrona	1983[29]	Stein	1989[51]
	O'Hara	1984[18]		
	Kumar	1984[2]		
	Campbell	1991[11]		
Caesarian section	Fisher	1990[43]		
	Hannah	1992[46]		
Breast-feeding	Dennerstein	1989[1]	Kumar	1984[2]
	Alder	1983[45]	Hannah	1992[46]

Table 5.2 Obstetric and gynaecological factors associated with risk of PND

depression before the onset of PND. Several surveys[22,23,30,52] found a positive correlation between neurotic personality in pregnancy and PND. However, we know that many women with PND have already suffered from depressive symptoms during the pregnancy. Their current state almost certainly affected the results of personality testing, and no firm conclusions can be drawn. A similar criticism can be directed at the conclusion that high interpersonal sensitivity increases the risk of postnatal depression at three months by a factor of 11[52].

Some psychologists have related depression to the individual's tendency to be angry with herself. One study looking at this factor showed just the contrary, that women who blamed others were more likely to be depressed postpartum, as were those who felt that they had little control over their own lives[29].

Psychiatric Symptoms During Pregnancy

Several studies have related high levels of anxiety during pregnancy to PND[3,10,23,53], but, perhaps more significantly, one found it to correlate with a pre-pregnant rating of 'always been a worrier'[22].

The majority of studies have shown a considerable proportion of women whose depression appears to be continuous throughout pregnancy and into the puerperium[1,10,17,31,36]. However, two other careful studies showed no relationship between antenatal and postnatal depression[2,22].

Previous Personal or Family History of Psychiatric Illness

Perhaps the most important indicator of vulnerability is a history of previous depressive illness, whether postnatal or not. The incidence of previous psychiatric contact in a group of young healthy women is likely to be low, and varies in different studies from 6% to 14%. In spite of this generally low incidence, one study showed that 60% of those depressed at six weeks postpartum had a previous history of psychiatric consultation[23]. Several others showed that there was a significantly increased number who had previously consulted the family doctor for psychiatric problems, usually depression[10,39,46]. One multinational study even found the risk higher in women who had previously experienced premenstrual mood disorder[1], although current depression may have coloured their recollection of PMS (see Case Study 5.3).

The risk of recurrence of postnatal depressive disorder is variously reported at levels from 25% to 75%[54,55]. Dalton's figures[54] are particularly confusing, suggesting that previous PND is not a good predictor of subsequent illness, but that the untreated recurrence rate is 68%. One study found that women without previous PND had low depression scores which did not relate to parity, but those with previous PND had high post-partum depression scores, which were especially marked in the group with three or more children[8]. This suggests that the previous illness(es) may have been partially unresolved. Forty per cent of their postnatally depressed women had had a previous episode of PND.

Other factors appear to combine with previous PND in a synergistic manner. For example, the recollection of low mood after a previous birth together with an EPDS score of 13 or more on the fifth postpartum day increased the risk of PND 85-fold[46].

Psychiatric illness in family members is more difficult to establish and to quantify. An American study comparing women with and without PND found that three times as many women with PND had at least one first degree relative who had been depressed[24]. There is some indication that previous depressive illness in the woman's mother during her own childhood may have a part to play, although this may be an environmental rather than a genetic factor[38].

Clinically, it is common to find women with PND reporting female relatives with a similar condition, and, in such families, there is also a higher incidence of other 'hormonally related' disorders such as PMS or depression related to oral contraception and the menopause. This has not been substantiated in research studies as yet.

The 'Blues'

Almost all research studies have shown a relationship between the 'blues' and later postnatal depression. Symptom scores and EPDS scores during the first 14 days postpartum, together with other aspects of personal history and current social situation are good predictors of later postnatal mood[14,22,46,56,57]. Approximately half the women with severe 'blues' continue to be depressed later in the puerperium. About one-third of women still depressed one year after the birth report that the illness began very soon after delivery.

Conclusion

Thus, even if risk factors have been missed in pregnancy, an assessment early in the puerperium will identify many of the women vulnerable to later and more chronic postnatal depression. This would allow the midwife or health visitor to be alerted to potential problems at a stage when added support might be protective. Research studies on personality and psychiatric factors associated with PND are cited in Table 5.3.

Biological Factors Associated with PND

It is clear that profound and rapid hormonal and biochemical changes occur in all postpartum women, whilst only some experience mood disorder. It seems more likely that these women have an abnormal reaction to one or more of these changes, rather than the changes themselves being responsible.

Few studies have examined hormones and other biochemical factors late in the puerperium, or in relation to postnatal depression alone; most have been concerned with the 'blues' or puerperal psychosis.

Since the maximum hormonal and biochemical changes occur early in the puerperium, and postnatal depression is generally of gradual onset at a later date, there is less reason to suppose that endocrine factors are implicated. As already shown, there are vast differences in individual vulnerability and profound changes in marital and family dynamics during the first postnatal year; these may be more relevant than hormonal factors to the onset of depression.

Oestrogen

An investigation of the relationship between breast-feeding and depression showed that those who were least likely to be

Risk factor	Studies finding increased risk		Studies finding no increased risk	
'Neurotic' personality	Watson	1984[23]	Kumar	1984[2]
	Cox	1982[22]		
	Pitt	1968[30]		
	Boyce	1991[52]		
Previous PMS	Dennerstein	1989[1]		
	Anzalone	1977[32]		
Previous psychiatric illness	Elliott	1984[41]	Kumar	1984[2]
	Paykel	1980[4]	Pitt	1968[30]
	O'Hara	1984[18]	Blair	1970[33]
	Playfair	1981[10]		
Previous PND	Hannah	1992[46]		
	Braverman	1978[39]		
	Playfair	1981[10]		
Family history of psychiatric illness	Elliott	1984[41]	Kumar	1984[2]
	O'Hara	1984[18]		
	Watson	1984[23]		
Depression in pregnancy	Robinson	1989[36]	Kumar	1984[2]
	Green	1990[31]	Cox	1982[22]
	Dennerstein	1989[1]		
	Pfost	1990[17]		
	Playfair	1981[10]		
Anxiety in pregnancy	Hayworth	1980[3]	Kumar	1984[2]
	Meares	1976[53]	Cox	1982[22]
	Watson	1984[23]		
	Playfair	1981[10]		
Postnatal 'blues'	Dalton	1971[54]	Kumar	1984[2]
	Paykel	1980[4]		
	Cox	1982[22]		
	Garvey	1983[55]		
	Hannah	1992[46]		
	Dennerstein	1989[1]		

As with Tables 5.1 and 5.2, the apparent discrepancies between research findings are due to differences in criteria for PND, together with the fact that most studies are carried out on a sample size of approximately 100–200 women. Since the incidence is only in the order of 10–20%, the actual number of sufferers is small, and the correlation of PND with predisposing factors open to inaccuracies.

Table 5.3 Personality and psychiatric factors associated with PND

depressed were those who were most likely to have normal levels of endogenous hormones[45]. They were neither totally breast-feeding, nor taking the oral contraceptive pill. Thus, ovarian suppression from whatever cause seems likely to be related to depression in vulnerable women.

Lower serum oestradiol levels were found in a group of women with high scores on the EPDS at one month postpartum[58], but two other studies found no difference in oestrogen levels between depressed and non-depressed subjects[59,60]. In spite of these equivocal findings, there is encouraging evidence that oestradiol skin patches can improve severe postnatal depression[61].

Clinically, it is not uncommon to find women developing postnatal depressive symptoms at the time of restarting the oral contraceptive pill, or beginning to improve from their postnatal depression when normal menstruation returns.

Progesterone

There are confusing results from a study of salivary hormones and mood[59]. In bottle-feeders, progesterone was positively associated with depression, but the reverse was true for breast-feeding mothers.

The use of progesterone by injection has been advocated both for the treatment and for the prevention of postnatal depression in vulnerable women[62]. This may well be due to the fact that progesterone is a mild sedative, or alternatively, it could be a placebo response. The only controlled trial, in a small number of patients, showed that progesterone was no more effective than placebo[63].

Androgens

All women produce significant levels of androgens from the ovary and adrenal gland. Some aspects of puerperal mood, such as low mood, sadness and fatigue, have been found to be associated with low levels of androgens at four months postpartum[64].

Cortisol

We know that cortisol levels decline dramatically from late pregnancy to the early puerperium[65]. One early study treated depressed postnatal out-patients with a reducing dose of predni-solone over a three-to-four week period; there was more rapid improvement than those treated with psychotropic drugs alone[66]. This study has not been repeated or confirmed. The few studies that have been carried out find no convincing relationship between cortisol levels and PND[6,59,67].

The dexamethasone suppression test, which is often abnormal in depressed patients, has also been found to be abnormal in postnatal women[67], but this may well be due to changes in other parameters such as weight. It showed no correlation with depressed mood.

Interestingly, it has been found that higher serum cortisol levels postpartum are related to more affectionate and infant directed behaviour in new mothers[68].

Thyroid Hormone

One report shows that there was no difference in thyroid function one month after delivery between those with depression and those without[67]. However, we know that thyroid function changes considerably throughout pregnancy and the puerperium[70], and that 20% of women have mild postpartum thyroid dysfunction, usually hyperthyroidism, between one and four months, or hypothyroidism from four to eight months postpartum. Many of the cases of hypothyroidism have high levels of thyroid antibodies. One recent study[71] screened 100 postpartum women and found a clear association between disturbed thyroid dysfunction and depression. Another[72] found a correlation between thyroid antibodies and depression, irrespective of thyroid status.

Clinical experience shows that a small proportion of women referred for a psychiatric opinion for postnatal depression are actually suffering from thyroid insufficiency. It is always worth checking thyroid function in suspected PND.

Tyramine

Tyramine is an amino acid, present in a normal diet. It is thought to be involved in the biochemical changes associated with migraine. Patients prone to episodes of endogenous depression seem to absorb more and excrete less after an oral dose than patients without a depressive history. In one study this loading test did not distinguish those with postnatal depression from controls, suggesting a different biochemical vulnerability in postnatal women[73].

Tryptophan and Non-esterified Fatty Acids

Tryptophan is also an amino acid, and is a substrate for the production of serotonin, a potent neurotransmitter. Serotonin deficiency has been related to depression. One early study showed a relationship between low levels of free tryptophan and some features of depression. This was confirmed by other investigators[6,74,75] who showed that women with symptoms of the 'blues' had a later postpartum rise in serum tryptophan levels than the remainder. Women who sought help for mood problems within the first six months postnatally were also more likely to show a similar change. A later investigation by the

Hormonal or biochemical factor	Definite correlation		No correlation	
Oestrogen	Kelly	1992[58]	Gard	1986[76]
			Harris	1989[59]
			Nott	1976[60]
Progesterone			Gard	1986[76]
			Nott	1976[60]
Androgens	Alder	1983[45]		
Cortisol			Handley	1980[6]
			Greenwood	1984[68]
			Gard	1986[76]
			Harris	1989[59]
Thyroid	Harris	1989[59]	Grimmell	1965[69]
	Pop	1991[71]		
Tyramine			Glover	1992[73]
Tryptophan	Handley	1977[75]	Handley	1980[6]
	Stein	1976[74]		
Non-esterfied fatty acids	Gard	1986[76]		

Table 5.4 Hormonal and biochemical factors associated with PND

same workers[76] confirmed this, but also showed that the level of non-esterified fatty acids (which may affect the levels of free tryptophan in serum) were raised in postnatal depression. Tryptophan supplementation has not been shown to alleviate early postnatal mood change[77].

Research Findings

Studies concerning the association between PND and hormonal and biochemical factors are shown in Table 5.4.

Infant Factors Associated with PND

Not all babies are placid and easy to care for, and a difficult baby can be a major source of stress in the postpartum period. In some cases, there are obvious difficulties such as prematurity, jaundice, or congenital abnormality, but often, infant temperament seems equally important.

In the past, this has often been related to the mother's depression and anxiety. It was thought that her inconsistent and tentative handling led to the baby being demanding and difficult to comfort, but more recent studies have tried to separate out the two factors. Two recent studies[78,79] have related stress attributable to child care, an indirect measure of infant temperament, to postpartum depressive symptoms. It was shown that depressed and non-depressed mothers were similar in terms of social and marital support, and that neonatal complications accounted for 12% of the variability in depression scores[79]. The mothers' perception of their children as 'fussy, unadaptable and unpredictable' accounted for a further 5%. There was no independent rating of the children's behaviour, so the mothers' view may have been coloured by their depressive state. Whichever came first, there are important implications for the longer-term mother–child interaction, and later behavioural problems in the child.

Mothers of 'high risk' infants report higher levels of emotional distress, more anxiety about themselves and their babies, and more difficulty in expressing affection to the babies[79]. Depressive symptoms were found to correlate with the degree of neo-natal risk and dissatisfaction with social support from family and friends.

Many women with problems with bonding to their babies also suffer from postnatal depression, but which is cause and which effect in these cases is often difficult to establish.

Conclusions

In spite of the content of this chapter, it seems that childbirth is often a truly 'happy event'; nine out of 10 mothers will negotiate pregnancy and childbirth safely and well in both physical and emotional terms. The general consensus of opinion is that there is only a small increase in the incidence of depression in new mothers compared with women of similar age who are neither pregnant nor have had a baby within the previous 12 months. However, the onset of PND does not appear to be evenly spread over time, and seems to be concentrated within the first few weeks or months after childbirth.

Although the public perception of the cause of postnatal depression is a 'hormonal imbalance', there is little hard evidence that this is the case. In most cases, it appears to be a continuation of a mood disorder arising before conception, or during the pregnancy. It is certainly more common in those women with previous depressive illness or without a supportive partner, and in those with poor socio-economic resources or adverse life events in the months before or immediately after the birth. It may be more common and more prolonged in those lacking practical and emotional support from family and friends. The occurrence and severity of the 'blues' in the early puerperium can also be a warning sign of later depressive symptoms.

This does not mean that we can be complacent about PND. The rates of depression in women of this age group are unacceptably high in comparison with the general population, and may even represent a large pool of prolonged and untreated PND amongst the control sample. In addition, postnatal depression arises at a crucial and sensitive period for the family;

a time when both mother and father are struggling to adapt to multiple and complex changes in their life-style and relationship. If this critical period is not negotiated well, it may have profound and far-reaching effects on the closeness of the parental relationship, the emotional stability of other children and the development of the infant.

There are indications that a vulnerability to postnatal illness can be identified early in the pregnancy, and that antenatal education, support and counselling directed towards vulnerable women can be beneficial[80,81]. The cost of the physical care offered to pregnant and postnatal women is high, and is fully justified by the high standards of maternal and neonatal physical health that have been achieved. Perhaps equal attention should now be paid to the emotional health of pregnant and postpartum women so that pregnancy, childbirth and child care can be happy as well as healthy for a larger proportion of women.

Case Study 5.1

Jane was a 29-year-old state registered nurse whose second child had been born three months previously. The pregnancy had been planned and normal, and she had an uncomplicated delivery. She was devastated to discover that the baby had bilateral congenital dislocation of the hips, as had her first daughter, two years previously. Jane felt embarrassed and ashamed at having the baby in a cumbersome splint, and felt that she could not 'get close' to her.

She had been tearful, miserable, irritable and angry, and felt that she was not coping well with household chores. Her husband had been helpful at first, but had returned to a new job necessitating frequent trips abroad. Her mother lived near, and visited daily, but was somewhat dominant and intrusive, often criticizing Jane for having an untidy house, and for being irritable with her older child.

Jane was an only child, and described a reasonably happy middle-class childhood, although she felt that the family were over-concerned about achievement and appearances. She had been quite rebellious in her teens, performing badly at school, and leaving without qualifications because she became pregnant at 16 years, just before her leaving examination. Jane was very tearful when describing how her parents had insisted on a termination, making all the arrangements for her, and leaving her no choice. She had felt resentful about the circumstances of the actual procedure, and grieved that no-one had told her the sex of the baby, or explained about the method of its disposal. Jane understood her later nursing training as an attempt to resolve her guilt at 'destroying a life' by being involved in caring for others. She had married the father of her first pregnancy, and wanted to have a 'large, happy family'.

Jane showed some predisposing factors for PND:

- over-controlling and intrusive mother

- inadequate support from her husband

- previous unresolved grief about a termination

- distress at the baby's congenital abnormality

- feeling that the 'lost' child would have been perfect

- feeling that the congenital dislocation of the hip in both children was a 'punishment' for the previous termination of pregnancy

- feeling that she had 'failed' her family's insistence on high standards of achievement.

Jane made a good recovery after some counselling sessions.

Case Study 5.2

Karen's second child was born three months before she was referred with low mood, tearfulness, irritability, poor sleep pattern, and feelings of 'wanting to run away'.

The pregnancy had been planned and normal except for some sciatica. Labour was spontaneous and she had an epidural because of raised blood pressure. She felt that she was left alone a lot during the labour and became very exhausted. Her husband was anxious himself and not very supportive to her during the delivery. She finally had a forceps delivery for an undiagnosed occipitoposterior position, and the baby was distressed at birth, needing a few days in intensive care. Delivery was followed by a urinary infection, and her episiotomy was slow to heal. Karen had expected a normal labour, and felt herself to be a failure. She was weepy in hospital, but somewhat 'high' in mood on return home. This was followed by a gradual onset of loneliness and low mood six weeks after the birth.

Karen was a very intelligent, capable and organized woman, who worked as a highly paid computer programmer, and clearly valued herself for her achievements and success within her career. She returned to work soon after her first child, but was unsure whether she would be able to return now she had two children.

She had been depressed twice before in response to life changes, and her mother had a long history of depression and hypochondriasis dating from her own birth. She missed the stimulation of work and adult company during the day, and began to associate motherhood with low status, depression and ill health, fearing that she would have a protracted illness like her mother.

The predisposing factors in Karen were:

- poor mothering in her own childhood

- inadequate support from her husband in labour

- feeling that she had 'failed' her own high standards by having complications of delivery and in the puerperium

- loss of status and intellectual stimulation

- identification with her own depressed mother

- previous history of depression in response to life events

- family history of depression

- severe 'blues'.

Karen joined a mothers' therapy group, where she gained insight into her relationship with her own mother and her own need to separate from her through her own achievements. She negotiated a return to part-time work, and made a good recovery.

Case Study 5.3

Lynn was a 33-year-old housewife whose second son had been born five months previously. She had had a miscarriage in the previous year, and already had one son who was seven years old.

The pregnancy was planned and was normal throughout, and she had a normal delivery. She was initially disappointed to have another boy, and rejected the baby for several hours. The baby was fretful for the first four weeks, after which bonding seemed to improve, but he was then admitted to hospital for gastroenteritis, and Lynn found it hard to readjust to caring for him on discharge.

She gave a two-month history of feeling sad and irritable, especially with her older son. She had alarmed herself by wanting to hit him when he had been disobedient. She felt anxious and tense, with initial insomnia, loss of appetite and of weight. Her energy was poor, and her concentration impaired.

Lynn's father had died when she was two years old, and her mother currently worked abroad. She described multiple changes of home and of school as a child, and, as a result, achieved poorly and had no long-standing friends. She had a depressive illness soon after leaving school at age 15, needing antidepressant medication. She had numerous unskilled jobs and could never settle in any employment. There was also a history of moderately severe premenstrual symptoms.

Lynn married at age 21, and the marriage was happy at first. She did not suffer from depression after the birth of her first child. Her husband then had a long period of unemployment, followed by working in a music shop where he worked long hours with uncertain prospects. He also spent most evenings away from home playing in a band. The couple were new to the area, had no local friends, and considerable financial worries.

Lynn showed many of the predisposing factors for PND:

- recent move of house and area

- no local social support

- little support from partner

- financial worries

- loss of parent in childhood

- absent mother

- recent miscarriage

- previous depressive illness

- previous premenstrual syndrome

- fractious baby

- recent ill health of baby.

Lynn recovered following antidepressant medication, introduction to mother and toddler groups, and marital counselling sessions.

References

1. Dennerstein L, Lehert P and Riphagen F. (1989) Post-partum depression – risk factors. *Journal of Psychosomatic Obstetrics and Gynaecology.* **10** (Suppl): 53–65.

2. Kumar R and Robson KM. (1984) A prospective study of emotional disorders in childbearing women. *British Journal of Psychiatry.* **144**: 35–47.

3. Hayworth J, Little BC, Carter SB, et al. (1980) A predictive study of postpartum depression: Some predisposing characteristics. *British Journal of Medical Psychology.* **53**: 161–7.

4. Paykel ES, Emms EM, Fletcher J, et al. (1980) Life events and support in postnatal depression. *British Journal of Psychiatry.* **136**: 339–46.

5. Feggetter G, Cooper P and Gath D. (1981) Non-psychotic psychiatric disorders in women one year after childbirth. *Journal of Psychosomatic Research.* **25**: 369–72.

6. Handley SL, Dunn TL, Waldron G, et al. (1980) Tryptophan, cortisol and puerperal mood. *British Journal of Psychiatry.* **136**: 498–508.

7. Zajicek E and Wolkind S. (1978) Emotional difficulties in married women during and after the first pregnancy. *British Journal of Medical Psychology.* **51**: 379–85.

8. Murray D, Cox JL and Chapman G. (1994) A controlled study of the social correlates of postnatal depression. *British Journal of Psychiatry.* In press.

9. Ballard C, Davis R and Dean C. (1992) Postnatal depression in mothers and fathers. In: *Recent advances in childbearing and mental health.* Abstracts of the 6th International Conference of the Marcé Society. 26.

10. Playfair HR and Gowers JI. (1981) Depression following childbirth: A search for predictive signs. *Journal of the Royal College of General Practitioners.* **31**: 201–8.

11. Campbell SB and Cohn JF. (1991) Prevalence and correlates of postpartum depression in first-time mothers. *Journal of Abnormal Psychology.* **100**: 594–9.

12. Brown GW and Harris T. (1978) *Social origins of depression: A study of psychiatric disorder in women.* New York: The Free Press.

13. Harvey I and McGrath G. (1988) Psychiatric morbidity in spouses of women admitted to a mother and baby unit. *British Journal of Psychiatry.* **152**: 506–10.

14. Lovestone S. (1992) Postnatal psychiatric illness – the effect on men. In: *Recent advances in childbearing and mental health.* Abstracts of the 6th International Conference of the Marcé Society. 27.

15. Clarke M and Williams AJ. (1979) Depression in women after perinatal death. *Lancet.* **i**: 916–17.

16. Thorpe KJ, Dragonas T and Golding J. (1992) The effects of psychosocial factors on the mother's emotional well-being during early parenthood. *Journal of Reproductive and Infant Psychology.* **10**: 205–7.

17. Pfost KS, Stevens MJ and Lum CU. (1990) The relationship of demographic variables, antepartum depression and stress to postpartum depression. *Journal of Clinical Psychology.* **46**: 588–92.

18. O'Hara MW, Neunaber DJ and Zekoski EM. (1984) A prospective study of postpartum depression. *Journal of Abnormal Psychology.* **93**: 158–71.

19. Martin ME. (1977) A maternity hospital study of psychiatric illness associated with childbirth. *Irish Journal of Medical Science.* **146**: 239–44.

20. Ballinger CB. (1982) Emotional disturbances during pregnancy and following childbirth. *Journal of Psychosomatic Research.* **26**: 629–34.

21. Cutrona CE. (1982) Nonpsychotic postpartum depression: A review of recent research. *Clinical Psychology Review.* **2**: 487–503.

22. Cox JL, Connor YM and Kendell RE. (1982) Prospective study of the psychiatric disorders of childbirth. *British Journal of Psychiatry.* **140**: 111–17.

23. Watson JP, Elliott SA, Rugg AJ, *et al.* (1984) Psychiatric disorder in pregnancy and the first postnatal year. *British Journal of Psychiatry.* **144**: 453–62.

24. O'Hara MW. (1986) Social support, life events and depression during pregnancy and the puerperium. *Archives of General Psychiatry.* **43**: 569–73.

25. Nott PN. (1982) Psychiatric illness following childbirth in Southampton: A case register study. *Psychological Medicine.* **12**: 557–61.

26. Pound A, Cox A, Puckering C, *et al.* (1985) The impact of maternal depression on young children. In: (Stevenson JE, editor) *Recent research in developmental psychopathology.* Pergamon Press, Oxford. 3–10.

27. Martin CJ, Brown GW, Goldberg DP, *et al.* (1989) Psychosocial stress and puerperal depression. *Journal of Affective Disorders.* **16**: 283–93.

28. Cooper PJ, Campbell EA, Day A, *et al.* (1988) Non-psychotic psychiatric disorder after childbirth. *British Journal of Psychiatry.* **152**: 799–806.

29. Cutrona CE. (1983) Causal attributions and perinatal depression. *Journal of Abnormal Psychology.* **92**: 161–72.

30. Pitt B. (1968) Atypical depression following childbirth. *British Journal of Psychiatry.* **114**: 1325–35.

31. Green JM. (1990) Who is unhappy after childbirth?: Antenatal and intrapartum correlates from a prospective study. *Journal of Reproductive and Infant Psychology.* **8**: 175–83.

32. Anzalone MK. (1977) Postpartum depression and menstrual tension, life stress and marital adjustment. *Dissertation Abstracts International.* **37** (12-B, Part 1): 6297.

33. Blair RA, Gilmore JS, Playfair HR, *et al.* (1970) Puerperal depression: A study of predictive factors. *Journal of the Royal College of General Practitioners.* **19**: 22–5.

34. Hopkins J, Campbell SB and Marcus M. (1987) Role of infant-related stressors in postpartum depression. *Journal of Abnormal Psychology.* **96**: 237–41.

35. Murray L. (1992) The impact of postnatal depression on infant development. *Journal of Child Psychology and Psychiatry.* **33**: 543–61.

36. Robinson GE, Olmsted MP and Garner DM. (1989) Predictors of post-partum adjustment. *Acta Psychiatrica Scandinavica.* **80**: 561–5.

37. Oglethorpe RJL. (1989) Parenting after perinatal bereavement – a review of the literature. *Journal of Reproductive and Infant Psychology.* **7**: 227–44.

38. Nilsson A, Kaij L and Jacobson L. (1967) Postpartum mental disorder in an unselected sample. The importance of the unplanned pregnancy. *Journal of Psychosomatic Research.* **10**: 341–7.

39. Braverman J and Roux JF. (1978) Screening the patient at risk for postpartum depression. *Obstetrics and Gynecology.* **52**: 731–6.

40. Wolkind S and Zajicek E. (1978) Psychosocial correlates of nausea and vomiting in pregnancy. *Journal of Psychosomatic Research.* **22**: 1–5.

41. Elliott SA, Anderson M, Brough DI, *et al.* (1984) The relationship between obstetric outcome and psychological measures in pregnancy and the postnatal year. *Journal of Reproductive and Infant Psychology.* **2**: 18–32.

42. Oakley A and Rajan L. (1980) Obstetric technology and maternal wellbeing. *Journal of Reproductive and Infant Psychology.* **8**: 45–55.

43. Fisher JRW, Stanley RO and Burrows GD. (1990) Psychological adjustment to caesarian delivery: A review of the evidence. *Journal of Psychosomatic Obstetrics and Gynaecology.* **11**: 91–106.

44. Garel M, Lelong N and Kaminski M. (1987) Psychological consequences of caesarian childbirth in primiparas. *Journal of Psychosomatic Obstetrics and Gynaecology.* **6**: 271–82.

45. Alder E and Cox JL. (1983) Breast feeding and postnatal depression. *Journal of Psychosomatic Research.* **27**: 139–44.

46. Hannah P, Adams D, Lee A, *et al.* (1992) Links between early postpartum mood and post-natal depression. *British Journal of Psychiatry.* **160**: 777–80.

47. Bridge LR, Little BC, Hayworth J, *et al.* (1985) Psychometric antenatal predictors of postnatal depressed mood. *Journal of Psychosomatic Research.* **29**: 325–31.

48. Areskog B, Uddenberg N and Kiessler B. (1984) Postnatal emotional balance in women with and without a fear of childbirth. *Journal of Psychosomatic Research.* **28**: 213–20.

49. Dean C and Kendell RE. (1981) The symptomatology of puerperal illnesses. *British Journal of Psychiatry.* **139**: 128–33.

50. Gennaro S. (1988) Postpartal anxiety and depression in mothers of term and preterm infants. *Nursing Research.* **37**: 82–5.

51. Stein A, Cooper PJ, Campbell EA, *et al.* (1989) Social adversity and perinatal complications: Their relation to postnatal depression. *British Medical Journal.* **299**: 1073–4.

52. Boyce P, Parker G, Barnett B, *et al.* (1991) Personality as a vulnerability factor to depression. *British Journal of Psychiatry.* **159**: 106–14.

53. Meares R, Grimwade J and Wood C. (1976) A possible relationship between anxiety in pregnancy and puerperal depression. *Journal of Psychosomatic Research.* **20**: 605–10.

54. Dalton K. (1971) Prospective study into puerperal depression. *British Journal of Psychiatry.* **118**: 689–92.

55. Garvey MJ, Tuason VB, Lumry AE, *et al.* (1983) Occurrence of depression in the postpartum state. *Journal of Affective Disorders.* **5**: 97–101.

56. Kendell RE, McGuire RJ, Connor Y, *et al.* (1981) Mood changes in the first three weeks after childbirth. *Journal of Affective Disorders.* **3**: 317–26.

57. Hapgood CC, Elkind GS, Wright JJ. (1988) Maternity blues phenomena and relationship to later postpartum depression. *Australian and New Zealand Journal of Psychiatry.* **22**: 299–306.

58. Kelly A and Deakin JFW. (1992) Psychosocial and biological predictors of early postnatal depression. In: *Recent advances in childbearing and mental health*. Abstracts of the 6th International Conference of the Marcé Society.

59. Harris B, Johns S, Fung H, *et al.* (1989) The hormonal environment of postnatal depression. *British Journal of Psychiatry.* **154**: 660–7.

60. Nott PN, Franklin M, Armitage C, *et al.* (1976) Hormonal changes in mood in the puerperium. *British Journal of Psychiatry.* **128**: 379–83.

61. Henderson AF, Gregoire AJP, Kumar R, *et al.* (1991) Treatment of severe postnatal depression with oestradiol skin patches. *Lancet.* **338**: 816–7.

62. Dalton K. (1985) Progesterone prophylaxis used successfully in postnatal depression. *Practitioner.* **229**: 507–8.

63. Van der Meer YG, Loendersloot EW and Van Loenen AC. (1984) The effect of high dose progesterone in postpartum depression. *Journal of Psychosomatic Obstetrics and Gynaecology.* **3**: 67–8.

64. Alder EM, Cook A, Davidson D, *et al.* (1986) Hormones, mood and sexuality in lactating women. *British Journal of Psychiatry.* **148**: 74–9.

65. Smith R, Cubis J, Brinsmead M, *et al.* (1990) Mood changes, obstetric experience and alterations in plasma cortisol, beta-endorphin and corticotrophin releasing hormone during pregnancy and the puerperium. *Journal of Psychosomatic Research.* **34**: 53–69.

66. Railton I. (1961) The use of corticoids in postpartum depression. *Journal of The American Medical Women's Association.* **16**: 450–2.

67. Brinsmead M. (1985) Peripartum concentrations of beta-endorphin and cortisol and maternal mood state. *Australian and New Zealand Journal of Obstetrics and Gynaecology.* **25**: 194–7.

68. Greenwood J and Parker G. (1984) The dexamethasone test in the puerperium. *Australian and New Zealand Journal of Psychiatry.* **18**: 282–4.

69. Grimmell K and Larsen VL. (1965) Postpartum depressive psychiatric symptoms and thyroid activity. *Journal of the American Medical Women's Association.* **20**: 542–6.

70. Fung HYM, Kologlu M, Collison K, *et al.* (1988) Postpartum thyroid dysfunction in Mid-Glamorgan. *British Medical Journal.* **296**: 241–4.

71. Pop VJM, de Rooy HAM, Vader HL, *et al.* (1991) Postpartum thyroid function and depression in an unselected sample. *New England Journal of Medicine.* **324**: 1815–6.

72. Harris B, Othman S, Davies JA, *et al.* (1992) Association between postpartum thyroid dysfunction, thyroid antibodies and depression. *British Medical Journal.* **305**: 152–6.

73. Glover V. (1992) How biochemical is postnatal depression? *Progress in Neuropsychopharmacology and Biological Psychiatry.* **16**: 605–15.

74. Stein G, Milton F, Bebbington P, *et al.* (1976) Relationship between mood disturbance and free and total plasma tryptophan in postpartum women. *British Medical Journal.* **ii**: 457–9.

75. Handley SL, Dunn DL, Baker JM, *et al.* (1977) Mood changes in the puerperium and plasma tryptophan and cortisol concentrations. *British Medical Journal.* **ii**: 18–22.

76. Gard PR, Handley SL, Parsons AD, *et al.* (1986) A multivariate investigation of postpartum mood disturbance. *British Journal of Psychiatry.* **148**: 567–75.

77. Harris B. (1980) Prospective trial of L-tryptophan in maternity blues. *British Journal of Psychiatry.* **137**: 233–5.

78. Bennett DE and Slade P. Infants born at risk: Consequences for postpartum adjustment. *British Journal of Medical Psychology.* **64**: 159–72.

79. Hopkins J, Campbell SB and Marcus M. (1987) Role of infant-related stressors in postpartum depression. *Journal of Abnormal Psychology.* **96**: 237–41.

80. Quinton C and Riley D. (1993) Does psychiatric intervention in pregnancy prevent postnatal depression? *Auditorium.* **2**: 58–63.

81. Leverton TJ and Elliott SA. (1989) Transition to parenthood groups: A preventive intervention for postnatal depression? In: (van Hall EV and Everaerd W, editors.) *The free woman. Women's health in the 1990s.* Parthenon, Carnforth, Lancs. 479–86.

6 Puerperal Psychosis

Incidence

Puerperal psychosis is the most severe and, fortunately, the most rare form of postnatal psychiatric disorder, occurring in approximately one in 500 newly delivered mothers. The illness is generally so severe that most of these women require admission to hospital, whereas few with postnatal depression do. Hospital admission figures therefore give a reasonable indication of the incidence of puerperal psychosis.

Table 6.1 shows the remarkable constancy of the figures for hospital admissions in relation to the number of deliveries in a representative sample of studies in various countries over a period of nearly 150 years.

Author	Year	Country	No. per 1000 live births
Marcé	1858[1]	France	2.2
Boyd	1942[2]	USA	2.5
Kline	1955[3]	USA	2.5
Hemphill	1956[4]	Great Britain	1.4
Ryle	1961[5]	Great Britain	1.9
Osterman	1963[6]	Sweden	1.0
Tod	1964[7]	Great Britain	2.9
Daniels	1964[8]	USA	1.0
Paffenbarger	1964[9]	USA	1.9
Karacan	1970[10]	USA	1.7–5.0
Brew and Seidenberg	1950[11]	USA	1.0–2.0
Grundy	1975[12]	Great Britain	1.9
Kendell	1981[13]	Great Britain	2.0

Table 6.1 Incidence of hospital admissions for puerperal psychiatric disorder

Time of Onset

The onset is usually early, commonly within the first two weeks after delivery, and almost always during the first month postpartum.

There is some evidence that manic puerperal illnesses present earlier in the puerperium than major depressive illnesses[14], and clinically it is common to find that the latter were preceded by a brief period of elation.

Characteristically, the onset is after a 'latent' period of a few days, and this is a phenomenon also found in postoperative psychoses. The early stages may be mistaken for a severe episode of the 'blues', but the symptoms rapidly escalate rather than subside.

Characteristics

Opinion is divided about the classification of the illness, probably because sufferers are not a homogeneous group, and because research workers have imposed their own diagnostic 'set' on an illness which is characteristically mixed in symptomatology.

Confusion

Interestingly, many of the older authors made a diagnosis of 'toxic confusional state', since puerperal infections were common and the symptoms often include bewilderment and mental confusion, features normally found only in psychosis of organic origin. With the advent of antibiotics and better obstetric management, toxic states in the puerperium are rare, yet the incidence of puerperal psychosis has not diminished over time. It is very unlikely that the incidence of functional disorders has increased during the same period, so that 'confusional states' occurring in recent years in the absence of gross physical pathology may have been re-allocated into categories of functional psychosis, ignoring evidence which would suggest an organic origin.

In support of this view, there are many reports of mental confusion as an integral part of the syndrome. This is a symptom not normally associated with functional psychoses, and in other circumstances can lead to doubt about a firm diagnosis. One psychiatric textbook[15] states:

'... in the early stages of the illness, the clinical picture is often not typical. There are very often prodromal symptoms of insomnia, restlessness, depression and irritability, leading to euphoria, refusal of food and the expression of irrational ideas. Furthermore, clouding of consciousness, particularly early in the illness, occurs much more commonly than in non-puerperal functional psychoses.'

The American Psychiatric Association, in their quick reference guide to the third edition of the *Diagnostic and statistical manual*[16] give a useful flow chart of differential diagnosis of psychotic features. It suggests that psychotic features in the presence of 'known organic factors by history or medical laboratory examinations' should be given a diagnosis of organic delusional syndrome, hallucinosis or other organic brain syndrome. There is a theoretical case for considering the major hormonal and biochemical changes following childbirth to be such 'known organic factors'.

Mixed Symptomatology

Even when confusion and clouding of consciousness are less evident, the syndrome is often difficult to categorize. This may explain the wide discrepancy in diagnostic categories reported by different authors, and the fact that there is no consistent trend of diagnostic pattern over time (*see* Table 6.2). This extent of disagreement by skilled and experienced psychiatrists implies that the syndrome itself is both confused in symptomatology and confusing to those trying to make a diagnosis.

Many authors have noted the presence of schizophrenic-type symptoms in otherwise typical affective illnesses in puerperal women[17], and an affective component in puerperal schizophrenia. Schizo-affective illness is rarely diagnosed in general psychiatry. With the most rigorous scrutiny, only 4% of all

Author	Year	Schizophrenic (%)	Affective (%)	Schizo-affective (%)	Confusional state (%)
Esquirol	1845[26]	8	91	–	–
Runge	1911[27]	37	20	–	25
Gregory	1924[28]	16	45	–	28
Saunders	1929[29]	60	40	–	–
Karnosh	1937[30]	10	43	–	45
Boyd	1942[2]	18	31	–	29
Jacobs	1943[31]	3	43	18	30
McNair	1952[32]	–	–	100	–
Foundeur	1957[33]	50	25	–	–
Martin	1958[34]	20	37	38	3
Madden	1958[35]	71	5	–	–
Pugh	1963[36]	50	31	–	19
Prothero	1969[24]	28	67	12	5
Paul	1974[37]	13	74	6	–
Dean	1981[19]	1	82	2	–
Katona	1982[20]	–	89	28	–
Brockington	1988[38]	24	43	26	–
Kompenhouwer	1991[39]	4.4	22		

Table 6.2 Diagnostic categories of puerperal psychosis

psychoses can be given this diagnosis[18]. The high incidence of schizo-affective diagnoses in the reports in Table 6.2 confirms the clinical impression that puerperal illnesses are characterized by a simultaneous occurrence or rapid fluctuation of affective and schizophrenic symptoms, and that some, at least, differ in material ways from psychoses occurring at other times.

One careful comparison of puerperal psychotic women with non-puerperal psychotic controls[19] concluded that the puerperal major depressives were 'more deluded and hallucinated, agitated, labile and disorientated than non-puerperal psychotic patients.' And another[20] found that 'Puerperal subjects were strikingly more often deluded than controls, and puerperal depressives were also more labile in mood.' A comparison of puerperal manic patients with a matched non-puerperal control group showed that the puerperal manics had a higher incidence of schizophrenic symptoms[17].

However, in other cases, we know that a previous history of manic depressive or schizo-affective disorder in the woman herself increases the risk of puerperal psychosis by a factor of at least 100, possibly more[21,22], and those with a family history of manic-depressive illness also run a higher risk than the population at large[23-25]. It seems most likely that puerperal illness is a variant of manic-depressive illness, changed in some way by the puerperal state.

Psychiatrists should note that whatever the clinical coding given to puerperal patients, a further coding should be made under ICD 10, Category O99.3 – 'Mental disorders and diseases of the nervous system complicating pregnancy, childbirth and the puerperium' – so that future researchers can easily identify puerperal admissions. If the psychosis is absolutely unclassifiable under the normal diagnostic criteria, then ICD 10, Code F53.1 covers 'severe mental and behavioural disorders associated with the puerperium, not elsewhere classified'.

From Table 6.2 it will be seen that the proportion of schizophrenic diagnoses varies from 0 to 71%, and of affective diagnoses from 0 to 91%. That this amount of diagnostic confusion could occur in cases studied sufficiently thoroughly to warrant publication suggests that the illness itself is atypical and presents a confusing picture. It would appear that, in many cases, schizophrenic and affective symptoms occur simultaneously or in rapid succession, and that the final disposal into diagnostic category is somewhat arbitrary, depending on the predominance of each type of symptomatology and the diagnostic orientation of the clinician. One school of thought[40] suggests that the illness should be described as a spectrum psychosis, showing signs of affective, schizophrenic and organic features, with rapid variation of symptoms. These authors liken this to the organic psychosis produced by the administration of steroids.

Another possible explanation of such diagnostic confusion is that puerperal psychoses are a heterogeneous group of illnesses made up from:

- women with a pre-existing schizophrenic illness who relapse in the puerperium

- women with a genetic predisposition to schizophrenia, whose first episode occurs in the puerperium

- women with a pre-existing affective psychosis who relapse in the puerperium

- women with a genetic predisposition to affective psychosis whose first episode occurs in the puerperium, and who may or may not go on to have non-puerperal episodes later

- women with no personal or genetic predisposition who only have puerperal illnesses.

Thus it is possible that women in the first four groups will have puerperal illnesses of the type to which they are predisposed by virtue of their personal or family history, whereas those in the last group may have illnesses of an 'organic' type related to the enormous hormonal and biochemical changes of the early puerperium, or, more likely, to an over-sensitivity to such changes, since the vast majority of women negotiate them without becoming mentally ill.

Clinical Picture

In the face of the diversity already referred to, it is difficult to give a 'typical' picture. However, some of the prominent and more common features are described below.

Clinically, these women usually present within the first two weeks postpartum with a history of sleep disturbance and a confusing mixture of symptoms. By definition, they have no insight into the fact that they are mentally ill. The typical patient is commonly restless, distractible, over-active and over-talkative, with racing thoughts and 'flight of ideas'. She may have grandiose ideas, and be irritable and even violent if these are thwarted.

> A patient seen at home, had turned the house upside down attempting to pack to go to Australia with her 8-day-old baby. She could give no good reason for wanting to do this. She was violent to her husband, accusing him of hiding her passport. At times she tried to breast-feed the baby, but was so distractible that after a few seconds, she would get up from her chair forgetting that the baby was still attached to the breast.

Depressive delusions, often about the baby, are common. The mother may believe that the baby is dead, deformed, or even that she is still pregnant. Characteristically, there is a pre-occupation with the contrast between good and evil. She may believe that the baby is evil – that it is able to harm her – or that others have evil intent towards her.

> One woman said that her baby's eyes changed colour when he looked at her, and that he was really the child of the devil. She constantly felt his forehead, and was convinced that he was growing horns.

She may hear voices commenting, usually critically, on her competence with the baby, or telling her to act in certain ways.

> Another saw a bright light, and heard a voice telling her that her baby was the son of God – and that she too had the power to save the world. She wanted to contact politicians to tell them how to prevent war and famine.

She may refuse food, believing that she does not need it, or that it is harmful. There may be paranoid beliefs about relatives or staff.

> A patient was convinced that her ex-husband, who had been violent towards her, was out of prison and hiding in the hospital ready to attack her again. She could not be reassured, even by speaking to the prison authorities. She said that she 'knew' he was there because she had seen a blue balloon on the ward.

Mood is often variable from hour to hour, changing from tearfulness and self-reproach to excitement and overactivity. When the mood is consistently depressed, there is often a history of elation earlier in the puerperium. There may also be bewilderment and disorientation in time, place and person. She may fail to recognize family members, and may not realize that she is in hospital. There is often later partial or complete amnesia for the period of illness.

Course and Prognosis

Early Outcome

In view of the differences in timing and type of illness described above, it is not surprising that reports of the outcome of puerperal psychosis are equally different. There is little point in looking at the overall prognosis and recurrence rate when all puerperal psychoses are treated as an entity. We should have more useful information to give to patients about their current illness and future risk if we divided the illnesses into the five groups already described on page 111.

A crude indication of outcome which is easily measured is the length of hospital admission. Table 6.3 gives a summary of published figures over recent years with an earlier paper for comparison.

In all comparisons of puerperal with non-puerperal women, the puerperal patients appear to recover more quickly. In individual patients, there appears to be a tendency to premenstrual relapse of symptoms for some time after the original illness.

It is also clear that women with affective illness appear to make a quicker recovery than those showing schizophrenic features, and this good outcome is confirmed by longer-term

Author	Year	Mean length of admission (months)		
		Schizophrenic	Affective	Total
Strecker	1926[41]	96	8.0	–
Martin	1958[34]	3.0	1.4	–
Prothero	1969[24]	3.8	2.4	–
Silberman	1975[42]	–	–	3.5
da Silva	1981[43]	–	–	2.25
Meltzer	1985[44]	1.98	1.3	–
Riley	1986[45]	–	–	1.43

Table 6.3 Mean length of admission for puerperal patients

follow-up studies[24,43]. The majority of women make a full re-covery from the psychosis, with no residual problems, but an initial illness of schizophrenic type carries a poorer prognosis for long-term mental ill health and difficulties with child rearing[43].

Recurrence

The burning question for women and their partners after a puerperal psychotic episode is whether the illness will recur after a future pregnancy. In many cases this fear is enough to deter them from having further children. Factors influencing recurrence include:

Previous puerperal psychosis

The overall risk of a further puerperal episode after an initial puerperal psychosis has been calculated from a large series of research studies as 1 : 5, compared with 1 : 500 for those without a previous illness. However, recent studies have put the risk of recurrence much higher, possibly at 1 : 2[22,25].

One study compared puerperal mania with similar non-puerperal illnesses in women of similar age[17]. Only one of the puerperal patients was readmitted within three years with a second puerperal episode, whilst there were six non-puerperal recurrences in the control group.

The risk of recurrence for women with only puerperal illness appears to diminish with subsequent pregnancies and to be less than that for women having both puerperal and non-puerperal illnesses.

Previous non-puerperal illness
The risk of a puerperal episode in women with previous bipolar affective disorder has been reported as at least 1 : 3[21,46].

It has been shown that a short period of time between the previous affective illness and the pregnancy is also a potent predictor of puerperal illness. In one study of 33 women with previous bipolar disorder, the overall incidence of puerperal illness was 58%, but all of those with illnesses within the previous two years relapsed in the puerperium[47] (*see* Case Study 6.1).

Family history of psychiatric illness
Several family studies have attempted to study this aspect of puerperal psychosis. In general the incidence of affective illness in the families of those with affective puerperal psychosis does not differ from that in the families of non-puerperal patients with affective illness[23,25], although one study[25] found it to be 50% in the first degree relatives of puerperal patients compared with 30% in non-puerperal bipolar disorder. However, clearly, both figures are higher than those found in the general population. We can therefore conclude that a family history of affective illness is a potent risk factor.

Risk of Non-puerperal Recurrence

Overall, the risk of future non-puerperal episodes for these women appears to be high. One study with a follow-up period of 5–24 years found 65% with one or more subsequent non-puerperal episodes[48].

Management of Women 'At Risk'

Before embarking on a further pregnancy, the risk of puerperal recurrence should be estimated for each individual, bearing in mind the personal and family history. It is probably least in a previously stable woman with a negative family history, and a previous puerperal illness of non-specific type with marked organic features.

However high the risk, it is possible to minimize the actual incidence of puerperal psychosis by reducing stressful events surrounding childbirth, and by the use of preventative medication. For example, lithium medication can be continued throughout the pregnancy[49] with a specialized scan at 16 weeks to exclude cardiac abnormality in the fetus, or begun soon after delivery[50]. The choice of action is determined by the risk of relapse when the patient stops lithium, together with any history suggesting a possible delay in conception. There is also current research into the protective effect of oestrogens given after delivery[47].

Causes

Effect of Parity

The risk in primiparae is approximately twice that in multiparae, and cannot be totally accounted for by the avoidance of further pregnancies in women who have already suffered from the illness, or by the primiparae being generally younger. Nevertheless, the illness is not exclusive to first pregnancies. There are many case reports of women suffering from puerperal psychosis for the first time after the second, third or fourth child.

Effect of Age

There is little indication that older or younger mothers are at a higher risk, but a large gap between the current and the previous pregnancy may be a factor[9].

Effect of Race

As already noted, there is good agreement about the incidence of puerperal psychosis in many studies carried out in all parts of the world, so that it is unlikely that race, religion or culture can be implicated. One British study[51] found an excess of recent immigrants, but this may be related to the added stress of adjustment in a strange culture rather than to a racial predisposition.

Marital Status

There is conflicting evidence of a small increase in incidence in unmarried mothers[13].

Social Class

There is little evidence that social class is a risk factor. The illness seems to occur equally across the social spectrum.

Complications of Pregnancy and Labour

These factors do not seem to have a significant effect. One study found a higher incidence of pre-eclamptic toxaemia, shorter gestation period and difficult labour[9], and one other[13] found an excess of caesarian sections in puerperal psychotic women. Although the numbers studied are small, there appears to be no increase with twin pregnancies.

Previous Psychiatric Illness

This is the most important predictive factor. As already noted, women with a history of manic-depressive illness run at least a 30% risk of a puerperal episode, possibly more.

Pre-existing schizophrenia may be exacerbated postpartum, but, more importantly, women with residual symptoms and poor social functioning after a pre-pregnancy episode find it difficult to cope with the demands of motherhood.

Previous puerperal psychosis also carries a risk of at least 30%, and if there have been non-puerperal episodes as well, the risk is higher still. All women with a previous history of this kind should be closely supervised during the pregnancy and puerperium so that symptoms can be identified at an early stage, and treatment given early to prevent escalation of the illness.

Genetic Factors

Most of the relevant research has compared the family histories of puerperal psychotic women with those of non-puerperal psychotics of similar age. There is no overall agreement between the studies, largely because of methodological differences. The only consensus is that there does not appear to be a hereditary factor related to 'pure' puerperal psychosis, and that the majority of affected relatives suffer from affective disorder.

However, there is an increased incidence of psychiatric illness in the first degree relatives of those women with puerperal psychosis when compared with the general population[23,25,49] (*see* Table 6.4). Only one study has looked at the incidence of mental illness in subsequent generations. This found an increase in mental illness in the children of women with puerperal psychosis, but no such increase in the grandchildren[52].

| | | Percentage of first degree relatives with psychiatric illness | |
| | | --- | --- |
Author	Year	Puerperal psychotic patients	Manic or manic-depressive patients
Cruikshank	1940[53]	30	–
		22[a]	–
		42[b]	–
McNair	1952[32]	30	–
Hemphill	1956[4]	14	–
Seager	1960[54]	30	–
Osterman	1963[6]	65	–
Paul	1974[37]	17	–
Kadrmas	1979[17]	19	38
Schopf	1985[48]	2[c]	–
		15.2[d]	–
Dean	1989[25]	19.9[c]	–
		20.2[d]	9.9[d]

[a]Toxic states.
[b]Manic-depressive.
[c]Patients with only puerperal illness.
[d]Patients with puerperal and non-puerperal episodes.

Table 6.4 Psychiatric illness in first degree relatives

Hormonal and Biochemical Factors

Puerperal psychosis would seem to be an ideal condition for research in that vulnerable individuals can be identified, and the time of onset of the illness predicted with some accuracy, so that prospective studies of hormonal and biochemical change can be carried out. Sadly, research findings are disappointing. There may be many reasons for this.

- Important findings have been diluted by including all puerperal patients who may be members of a heterogeneous group. It might be more illuminating to consider hormone and biochemical changes only in those women without a genetic predisposition to psychiatric illness.

- The incidence is so low that it is difficult to accumulate a large enough series of cases in any one centre.

- Hormone assays are expensive and complicated, and repeated blood sampling is unacceptable to many puerperal women.

- The hormonal differences between psychotic and non-psychotic women may be trivial in comparison with the massive changes occurring in all postpartum women.

- Only a small proportion of most hormones is free and active; the remainder is bound to protein molecules. There are profound changes in blood volume and protein levels in pregnancy and the early puerperium. These may affect the active fraction of hormones in unpredictable ways. Estimation of total hormone levels is therefore unhelpful.

- Many hormones have a marked variation in levels during the 24-hour day, and some are even pulsatile in secretion. Individual assessments of hormone levels may therefore be misleading.

- It is more likely that the balance between various hormones is more important than any single hormone level.

- There is increasing evidence that receptor sensitivity is a more accurate marker of hormone and neurotransmitter activity.

• Most neurotransmitter research has been done on platelets, and these do not necessarily give an accurate reflection of changes within the central nervous system.

Oestrogen

Total oestradiol levels increase during the course of pregnancy, reaching up to 200 times the normal levels occurring in the second half of the menstrual cycle[55]. Post-delivery there is a dramatic fall in level over the first 48 hours, reaching the lowest levels at one week postpartum[56,57]. There may also be a significant drop in pregnancy related protein, affecting the amount of free oestradiol in the serum[58].

There is contradictory evidence regarding oestrogen in relation to puerperal disorders. One study found that pre-delivery oestradiol concentrations were higher in those with irritable mood at 10 days postpartum[57], but several others have found no correlation of levels with mood[59-62]. Total serum levels are probably unhelpful, since 98% is protein bound and inactive. However, one study that measured levels in saliva, which more accurately reflects the unbound fraction, found that levels were high on days that symptoms occurred[63].

The indirect effects of oestrogen acting on neurotransmitters and peptides is probably more relevant. Very recent work has shown that there is an increase in dopamine receptor sensitivity in women who develop puerperal psychosis, and that this may be a response to oestrogen withdrawal[47].

Progesterone

There is conflicting evidence about the effect of progesterone levels on postnatal mood. One study found that the greatest drop in progesterone from pre- to postpartum was associated with low mood at 10 days[57], but this was not confirmed by other workers[59,62,64]. In spite of some early work suggesting that progesterone given postpartum could prevent depressive symptoms[65,66] there is no evidence to correlate progesterone levels with psychotic symptoms. Indeed one study reported unsuccessful attempts to treat three puerperal psychotic patients with progesterone[67].

Cortisol

As with ovarian steroids, there is a large increase in serum levels of cortisol during pregnancy with a precipitous postpartum fall[57,58]. An early study compared puerperal psychosis with the steroid withdrawal syndrome, and had some success in treating women with decreasing doses of prednisolone[69]. More recent evidence has been conflicting, some workers finding elevated cortisol levels to correlate with elated mood in the first postpartum week[69,71], and others finding high levels present in association with low mood[72]. However, there are difficulties in interpreting the results, since much of the hormone is bound to protein, and there is a large variation in cortisol levels throughout the day. There is some evidence that this periodicity is disturbed in severe depression[73], but no convincing evidence that it is implicated in puerperal psychosis. As with oestrogen, the indirect effects may be more important.

Thyroid

There are profound changes in thyroid parameters in all women during pregnancy and the first postpartum year[74], but minimal evidence to correlate these changes with puerperal psychosis. A careful study of puerperal psychotic women showed that all the thyroid function tests were within normal limits[75]. However, the free thyroxine index was significantly higher and the thyroid stimulating hormone (TSH) level lower than those of a postpartum control group. The difference in TSH was especially marked in the group with affective disorders. Other workers have shown that T_3 levels in women with major depression at one month postpartum were lower than in controls[72].

Prolactin

Prolactin increases in late pregnancy and falls postpartum, with surges related to breast-feeding[56]. There is one report of a correlation between basal prolactin levels and depression, anxiety and tension in the first postpartum week[76], but there is no confirmation of these findings by other research workers[57,62].

Oxytocin

Oxytocin levels in serum rise during pregnancy and this hormone has a role in initiating uterine contractions and the milk ejection reflex postpartum. Higher levels of oxytocin following electroconvulsive therapy (ECT) have correlated with clinical response[77], so that its effect may be implicated in mood disorder.

There is a single report of high serum oxytocinase levels in late pregnancy in a woman who later became psychotic[78]. This enzyme degrades oxytocin and may also have an effect on other peptides.

Peptide hormones

Beta-endorphin levels in serum rise towards the end of pregnancy, and reach a peak during labour. They then decline over the first postpartum week. Reduced β-endorphin levels have been implicated in the mood changes of the premenstrual syndrome, which has been likened to an opiate withdrawal syndrome. A similar mechanism is possible postpartum[79], but, since plasma β-endorphin does not cross the blood–brain barrier, the implication is still unclear. However, in one of the few studies on cerebrospinal fluid, high levels of an unusual opioid peptide were found in four of 11 puerperal psychotic patients, but in none of the normal lactating or non-lactating controls; the levels diminished on recovery[80].

Other biochemical factors

Alpha-adrenoceptor activity is reduced in depression and also postpartum as a result of oestrogen withdrawal. However, α-2-adrenoceptors in platelets showed higher binding capacity in women with the 'blues'[81].

Decreased β-receptor binding is found after antidepressant treatment or oestrogen administration. Postpartum oestrogen withdrawal may therefore reverse this change, and theoretically give rise to depressive symptoms.

There are no consistent findings in postnatal mood disorder regarding serotonin or monoamine oxidase, although both may be affected by oestrogen levels. However, recent work has shown that the onset of affective puerperal psychosis is associated with increased sensitivity of dopamine receptors in the brain[47]. As increased dopamine activity is known to be associated with psychotic illness, and neuroleptic drugs act by blocking dopamine, this is the most encouraging work so far.

One report suggests that high levels of ionized serum calcium are associated with psychosis in women with no previous personal or family history of psychosis – the 'organic' group described above[82]. Parathyroid hormone levels increase during pregnancy, but most of it is bound to protein, and therefore inactive. In the absence of pregnancy-related protein, there may be a rebound phenomenon. Some support for this is found in the fact that calcium-channel blockers have an antimanic and mood stabilizing effect[83,84].

Treatment

Where to Treat?

Hospitalization is usually necessary, although some services with good community support are able to care for these women in their own homes. If admission is required, it is obviously preferable to admit mother and baby together. This seems to decrease the mother's level of anxiety, keep her more in touch with reality, and preserve the bonding between mother and baby.

Other benefits of joint admission are a shorter stay in hospital, and a lower relapse rate (*see* Chapter 9 on service provision for more details on suitable accommodation and care).

Medication and Physical Treatment

Few authors comment in any systematic way on their methods of treatment, reflecting the difficulty of applying a standard regimen to such a polymorphous syndrome.

Treatment has to be symptomatic, and constantly has to weigh the benefits of medication against the risks to the baby of psychotropic drugs in breast milk. Clearly the continuity of breast-feeding is important, but may be unwise if large dosages of medication are needed[85].

Major tranquillizers are often indicated as a matter of urgency, to control disturbed and restless behaviour and to ensure sleep and adequate fluid intake. Haloperidol or its more recent derivatives are commonly used, and very large doses are often needed. Extrapyramidal side-effects seem to be more common and severe in these women, and additional medication to counter these is almost always required. They are also more susceptible to the hypotensive effects of medication[86], and daily sitting/standing blood pressures should be recorded. Where these drugs are ineffective in acceptable dosage, daily ECT can be helpful in controlling manic symptoms.

Where depressive symptoms are prominent, antidepressant medication can be added. The tricyclic group is tried and tested, but these drugs are slow to take effect and have side-effects that may be unacceptable to a mother caring for a child. The more recent 5-HT re-uptake inhibitors have less side-effects and work more quickly. However, we do not know the levels in breast milk of most of the newer antidepressants, and they are so far contra-indicated in breast-feeding mothers.

If the patient is suicidal, infanticidal or suffering from depressive delusions, or if there are concerns about dehydration from lack of fluid intake, then ECT should be considered. This often brings about rapid and dramatic improvement after only a few treatments. Many psychiatrists would consider ECT to be the first line of treatment for a mother with psychotic depression.

Both with antidepressant medication and with ECT, there is often a risk of precipitating manic symptoms in these patients, and the mental state should be carefully monitored, preferably in hospital.

Lithium is useful in two situations. First, in manic or schizo-manic patients, when the initial excitability has been controlled with major tranquillizers, it stabilizes mood, preventing a later 'down-swing' into depression. It is wise to be cautious about the combination of lithium with major tranquillizers; neuroleptic malignant syndrome also seems to be more common in the postpartum state. Early relapse is a problem in these women, and it is often sensible to continue lithium for 6–12 months following the initial illness (*see* Case Study 6.2). Secondly, in women with a history of manic or bipolar state, where the risk of a puerperal illness is high, it can be started during the third trimester or soon after delivery and is effective in reducing the recurrence of psychosis[50].

Other mood stabilizers such as carbamazepine, valproate or calcium-channel blockers may also be effective where lithium is contra-indicated or ineffective.

Hormonal Treatment

There are early reports of the effectiveness of oestrogen, but none of these were controlled trials. There is also concern about whether oestrogen might suppress lactation or predispose to thrombo-embolism. However, there has been renewed interest recently, and there is a current trial of oestrogen administered by skin patches together with an anticoagulant, in women at high risk for a postpartum recurrence of psychosis[87]. The preliminary results are encouraging.

No controlled trials of progesterone therapy have been carried out, but one author has claimed that it prevents early relapse of the illness[66].

One author noted that the symptoms resembled steroid withdrawal psychosis, and treated a small number of women with prednisolone[69]. This appeared to shorten the illness, or to prevent it in vulnerable women, but more rigorous trials with larger numbers are needed to confirm the findings.

Several psychiatrists have used thyroxine as an adjunct to treatment, chiefly in psychoses of late onset. There is little justification for this unless thyroid function tests are abnormal.

Vitamins

There is an isolated report of improvement with high doses of ascorbic acid[88], and another of eight cases treated with vitamin B_{12}[89]. Neither of these studies have been repeated or confirmed.

Practical Issues

These patients are a great worry to psychiatric nurses and doctors because they have to concern themselves with the safety and welfare of the baby as well as the patient herself. As already discussed, the illness tends to be fluctuant in intensity, and somewhat unpredictable in symptomatology, with a tendency to early relapse.

The mothers need a great deal of supervision and encouragement with coping with the baby, both whilst in hospital and after discharge. In spite of the concerns about admitting a baby with a psychotically disturbed mother, it has been shown that recovery is generally quicker in designated mother and baby units[90]. Careful supervision is of course needed, especially when the mother has delusional ideas about the child, but audits of such units[45,91] have shown that harm to the baby is rare, and is usually the result of neglect or carelessness rather than intent.

Assessments of the mother's maternal skills can be made with the aid of the Bethlem Mother–Infant Interaction Scale (*see* Appendix 6.1).

As the mother begins to improve, it is appropriate for her to have increasing periods of time at home, provided that suitable supervision can be provided by the relatives, or home carers. Unsupervised time with the baby in the home can be introduced in a gradual way as and when appropriate.

It is important to include the partner in explanation of the illness and its likely course and outcome. He may need a great deal of reassurance and support himself[92].

Each woman should have an individual plan of after-care made whilst she is still in hospital, and reviewed soon after discharge. This can include social support in the form of attendance at a family centre or mother and toddler groups, together with regular visits from the health visitor, and community psychiatric nurse. It is often difficult to strike the right balance between adequate and over-intrusive supervision, and the plan may need frequent revision.

Careful supervision from primary carers is necessary for a prolonged period in order to detect any signs of relapse. Medication and community support may continue to be needed for some months following the initial illness. A total care plan should include discussion of suitable contraception, especially if medication is continued, and also of the risks of a recurrence after a future pregnancy.

Case Study 6.1

Anne was an intelligent woman aged 27, who had experienced her first major depression at the age of 16, soon after the death of her mother. She was hospitalized for four months, and treated with ECT. Over the subsequent seven years she was readmitted with three further episodes of depression and one of mania. At age 23 she was established on lithium and remained well.

Anne's father and brother had also suffered major episodes of depression requiring admission to hospital.

Anne married aged 25, continuing to work as a personal assistant to the director of a company. Her husband was a computer programmer who had a rather rigid and obsessional personality.

She stopped taking lithium on medical advice before becoming pregnant. She remained well throughout the pregnancy, and had a normal delivery of a healthy boy.

Four days after the birth, she was noted to be agitated and restless after a poor night's sleep. Over the next few days, her mood became increasingly labile, and she was overactive, with some pressure of speech. Her conversation contained puns, spoonerisms and clang associations, and her noisy disinhibition embarrassed her husband. She was hostile towards him and the ward staff, and took no interest in the baby. She did not accept that she was ill.

Admission under Section 2 of the Mental Health Act was necessary, and her illness pursued a stormy course until she was re-established on lithium. There was one relapse when lithium was discontinued because of myxoedema, but it was re-started with the addition of thyroxine, and she has remained well since.

This case illustrates the case of a woman with a positive personal and family history of affective disorder, with a puerperal recurrence resembling her previous illness. Giving lithium in the third trimester, or immediately after the birth might have prevented or lessened the severity of the illness. She will be at approximately 1 : 2 risk of a recurrence after any future deliveries.

Case Study 6.2

Teresa was a 30-year-old woman who was admitted to hospital with her one-week-old baby because of inability to sleep and bizarre behaviour. She had had only one or two hours' sleep each night, and felt weak, tired and tense, afraid that burglars might break into the house. She was over-sensitive to noise, and somewhat over-talkative. She felt that she was going mad, and that her family doctor was evil because his eyes looked strange. There was a preoccupation with death, thinking that the children would die, and that she could see the devil.

She had no history of previous psychiatric illness, nor did her family of origin. She had always been a confident, cheerful woman who had been a successful hairdresser before the birth of her first child two years previously. There was no postnatal illness on that occasion.

Teresa had been upset a year earlier when her parents separated. The couple had also moved house just before the recent birth. On the day she went into labour, her husband was playing football, and sustained a severe facial fracture needing admission and operation. She was distressed that he could not be with her in labour, and frightened about possible permanent disfigurement.

She made a good recovery on antidepressant medication and halo-peridol. However, subsequent mood swings occurred, with depressive episodes related to the menstrual cycle. These were severe enough to affect her social functioning, and were controlled on lithium for six months. She has been free of medication since.

This illustrates a first episode in a woman of previously stable personality with no family history of psychiatric illness. It occurred in a setting of extreme social and emotional stress, and the illness itself was too prolonged to be diagnosed as a brief reactive psychosis. It was coded as an atypical psychosis in the puerperium. It remains to be seen whether the illness will recur in the future. Her chances of a puerperal recurrence are probably less than 1 : 5.

Appendix 6.1

BETHLEM MOTHER–INFANT INTERACTION SCALE

Patient's name: Date:

Baby's name: Nurse:

General Comments Relating to Previous Week

Mother's general health:

Baby's general health:

Any major events at home:

Any major events on ward:

Any changes of treatment plan:

Medication:

Other comments:

A. Eye Contact

0 – Mother generally seeks and maintains eye contact with baby in an appropriate way. Her regard and expression are responsive to baby's state (eg smiling, crying etc.).

1 – As above (0), but there are short breaks when mother may look away or seem not to focus on baby.

2 – As above (1) but breaks are longer and mother seems to initiate eye contact less often, giving the impression that there are times when she avoids looking at the baby, finds it uncomfortable to hold gaze, or is too distractible to do so.

3 – As above (2), but very little eye contact with baby.

4 – Not applicable: separated most of the time.

Comments:

B. Mood

0 – Generally comfortable, relaxed, caring, warm and sensitive to baby's mood and state. Able to tolerate baby's distress or irritability.

1 – As above (0), but punctuated by brief periods when effective responses to baby are inappropriate or lacking. Nevertheless, sensitive to baby much of the time.

2 – As above (1), but mother's mood dominates the interaction with the baby. Some of the time however, she is able to respond appropriately (eg successfully soothing baby or initiating play).

3 – Mostly out of harmony with baby. Mother's mood is not responsive to baby for more than a few moments at a time.

4 – Not applicable: separated most of the time.

Comments:

C. General Routine

0 – Well organized in relation to looking after baby (eg feeds and nappies generally prepared in good time; unflustered by unexpected minor problems; copes independently).

1 – As above (0), but occasional lapses which result in staff prompting or reminding mother. No serious difficulties.

2 – As above (1), but lapses more frequent and severe, so that staff often have to intervene and help.

3 – Very disorganized. Requires considerable intervention and help from staff every day.

4 – Not applicable: separated most of the time.

Comments:

D. Physical Risk to Baby

0 – Generally safe; no perceived risk to baby.

1 – Sometimes careless or neglectful, but quickly corrects or responds to risk.

2 – Unintentionally careless, rough or neglectful, thus putting baby in dangerous situations without awareness of risk.

3 – Threatens or definitely fears that she will harm the baby.

4 – Actual harm caused intentionally or unintentionally, or separated most of the time.

NB If there is a score of 2 or more on the 'Risk' scale, please describe in detail:

a. The nature of any incidents and indicate whether through neglect or intention.

b. If no actual incident, what the mother said to suggest risk.

c. Relevant aspects of mother's mental state (eg suicidal, manic, possible delusions incorporating baby).

E. Baby's Contribution to Interaction

0 – Healthy, alert, happy and responsive baby.

1 – Occasionally baby seems difficult or there is some health problem for most of the time.

2 – Clearly difficult or in poor health most of the time.

4 – Not applicable: separated most of the time.

NB If the baby is rated 1 or above, please indicate what the problem is in as much detail as possible.

Scores: A =

B =

C =

D =

E =

Total:

References

1. Marcé LV. (1858) *Traité de la folie des femmes enceintes, des nouvelles accouchées et des nourrices.* Baillière, Paris.

2. Boyd DA. (1942) Mental disorders associated with childbearing. *American Journal of Obstetrics and Gynecology.* **43**: 148–63.

3. Kline CL. (1955) Emotional illness associated with childbirth. *American Journal of Obstetrics and Gynecology.* **69**: 748–57.

4. Hemphill RE. (1956) Incidence and nature of puerperal psychiatric illness. *British Medical Journal.* **ii**: 1232–5.

5. Ryle A. (1961) The psychological disturbances associated with 345 pregnancies in 137 women. *Journal of Mental Science.* **107**: 279–86.

6. Osterman E. (1963) Les etats psychopathologiques du postpartum. *Acta Psychiatrica Scandinavica.* **39** (suppl.169): 190–3.

7. Tod EM. (1964) Puerperal depression: A prospective epidemiological study. *Lancet.* **ii**: 1264–6.

8. Daniels RS and Lessow H. (1964) Severe postpartum reactions. *Psychosomatics.* **5**: 21–6.

9. Paffenbarger RS. (1964) Epidemiological aspects of parapartum mental illness. *British Journal of Preventative and Social Medicine.* **18**: 189–95.

10. Karacan I and Williams RL. (1970) Current advances in theory and practice relating to postpartum syndromes. *Psychiatry in Medicine.* **1**: 307–28.

11. Brew MF and Seidenberg R. (1950) Psychotic reactions associated with pregnancy and childbirth. *Journal of Nervous and Mental Disease.* **111**: 408–23.

12. Grundy PF and Roberts CJ. (1975) Observations on the epidemiology of postpartum mental illness. *Psychological Medicine.* **5**: 286–90.

13. Kendell RE, Rennie D, Clarke JA, *et al.* (1981) The social and obstetric correlates of psychiatric admission in the puerperium. *Psychological Medicine.* 11: 341–50.

14. Brockington IF, Winokur G and Dean C. (1982) Puerperal psychosis. In: (Brockington IF and Kumar R, editors) *Motherhood and mental illness.* Academic Press, London, 37–69.

15. Granville Grossman K. (1971) Post-partum mental disorders. In: *Recent advances in psychiatry*: Vol. I. J & A Churchill, London, 266–311.

16. American Psychiatric Association. (1980) Quick reference to the diagnostic criteria from *Diagnostic and statistical manual of mental disorders*, 3rd edition. APA. Washington DC, 200–9.

17. Kadrmas A, Winokur G and Crowe R. (1979) Postpartum mania. *British Journal of Psychiatry.* 135: 551–5.

18. Brockington IF and Leff JP. (1979) Schizo-affective psychosis: Definitions and incidence. *Psychological Medicine.* 9: 91–9.

19. Dean C and Kendell RE. (1981) The symptomatology of puerperal illnesses. *British Journal of Psychiatry.* 139: 128–33.

20. Katona CLE. (1982) Puerperal mental illness: Comparisons with non-puerperal controls. *British Journal of Psychiatry.* 141: 447–52.

21. Bratfos O and Haug JO. (1966) Puerperal mental disorders in manic-depressive females. *Acta Psychiatrica Scandinavica.* 42: 285–94.

22. Marks MN, Wieck A, Seymour A, *et al.* (1992) Women whose mental illnesses recur after childbirth and partners' levels of expressed emotion during late pregnancy. *British Journal of Psychiatry.* 161: 211–16.

23. Whalley LJ, Roberts DF, Wentzel J, *et al.* (1982) Genetic factors in puerperal affective psychoses. *Acta Psychiatrica Scandinavica.* 65: 180–93.

24. Prothero C. (1969) Puerperal psychoses: A long-term study 1927–1961. *British Journal of Psychiatry.* 115: 9–30.

25. Dean C, Williams RJ and Brockington IF. (1989) Is puerperal psychosis the same as bipolar manic-depressive disorder? *Psychological Medicine.* 19: 637–47.

26. Esquirol E. (1845) *Mental maladies: A treatise on insanity.* Lea & Blanchard, Philadelphia.

27. Runge W. (1911) Die Generationpsychosen des Weißes. *Archives of Psychiatry.* **48**: 545–690.

28. Gregory MS. (1924) Mental diseases associated with childbearing. *American Journal of Obstetrics and Gynecology.* **8**: 420–30.

29. Saunders EB. (1929) Association of psychoses with the puerperium. *American Journal of Psychiatry.* **8**: 669–80.

30. Karnosh L and Hope J. (1937) Puerperal psychoses and their sequelae. *American Journal of Psychiatry.* **94**: 537–50.

31. Jacobs B. (1943) Aetiological factors and reaction types in psychoses following childbirth. *Journal of Mental Science.* **89**: 242–6.

32. McNair FE. (1952) Psychosis occurring postpartum. *Canadian Medical Association Journal.* **67**: 637–41.

33. Foundeur J, Fixsen C, Triebel WA, *et al.* (1957) Postpartum mental illness: A controlled study. *Archives of Neurology and Psychiatry.* **77**: 503–12.

34. Martin ME. (1958) Puerperal mental illness. *British Medical Journal.* **ii**: 773–7.

35. Madden JJ, Luhan JA, Tuteur W, *et al.* (1958) Characteristics of postpartum mental illness. *American Journal of Psychiatry.* **115**: 18–24.

36. Pugh TF, Jerath BK, Schmidt WM, *et al.* (1963) Rates of mental disease related to childbearing. *New England Journal of Medicine.* **268**: 1224–8.

37. Paul L. (1974) A study of puerperal psychosis. *Journal of the Indian Medical Association.* **63**: 84–9.

38. Brockington IF and Cox-Roper A. (1988) The nosology of puerperal psychosis. In: (Kumar R and Brockington IF, editors) *Motherhood and Mental Illness 2.* Wright, London, 1–16.

39. Klompenhouwer JL and van Hulst AM. (1991) Classification of postpartum psychosis: A study of 250 mother and baby admissions in the Netherlands. *Acta Psychiatrica Scandinavica.* **84**: 255–61.

40. Sneddon J and Kerry RJ. (1980) Puerperal psychosis. *British Journal of Psychiatry.* **136**: 520–4.

41. Strecker EA and Ebaugh FC. (1926) Psychoses occurring during the puerperium. *Archives of Neurology.* **15**: 239–52.

42. Silbermann RM. (1975) *CHAM, a classification of psychiatric states* [thesis]. Excerpta Medica, Amsterdam.

43. da Silva L and Johnstone EC. (1981) A follow-up study of severe puerperal psychiatric illness. *British Journal of Psychiatry.* **139**: 346–55.

44. Meltzer ES and Kumar R. (1985) Puerperal mental illness, clinical features and classification: A study of 142 mother and baby admissions. *British Journal of Psychiatry.* **147**: 647–54.

45. Riley DM. (1986) An audit of obstetric liaison psychiatry. *Journal of Reproductive and Infant Psychology.* **4**: 99–115.

46. Reich T and Winokur G. (1970) Postpartum psychoses in patients with manic depressive disease. *Journal of Nervous and Mental Disease.* **151**: 60–8.

47. Wieck A, Kumar R, Hirst AD, *et al.* (1991) Increased sensitivity of dopamine receptors and recurrence of affective psychosis after childbirth. *British Medical Journal.* **303**: 613–6.

48. Schopf J, Bryois C, Jonquiere M, *et al.* (1985) A family hereditary study of postpartum psychoses. *European Archives of Psychiatry and Neurological Science.* **235**: 164–70.

49. Schou M. (1990) Lithium treatment during pregnancy, delivery and lactation: An update. *Journal of Clinical Psychiatry.* **51**: 410–3.

50. Stewart DE, Klompenhouwer JL, Kendell RE, *et al.* (1991) Prophylactic lithium in puerperal psychosis. *British Journal of Psychiatry.* **158**: 393–7.

51. Kendell RE, Wainwright S, Hailey A, *et al.* (1976) The influence of childbirth on psychiatric morbidity. *Psychological Medicine.* **6**: 297–302.

52. Uddenberg N. (1974) Reproductive adaptation in mother and daughter. *Acta Psychiatrica Scandinavica.* Suppl. 254.

53. Cruikshank WH. (1940) Psychoses associated with pregnancy and the puerperium. *Canadian Medical Association Journal.* **43**: 571–6.

54. Seager CP. (1960) A controlled study of postpartum mental illness. *Journal of Mental Science.* **106**: 214–30.

55. Willcox DL, Yovich JL, McColm SC, *et al.* (1958) Changes in total and free concentrations of steroid hormones in the plasma of women throughout pregnancy. *Journal of Endocrinology.* **107**: 293–300.

56. Bonnar J, Franklin M, Nott PN, *et al.* (1975) Effect of breast feeding on pituitary–ovarian function after childbirth. *British Medical Journal.* **iv**: 82–4.

57. Nott PN, Franklin M, Armitage C, *et al.* (1976) Hormonal changes and mood in the puerperium. *British Journal of Psychiatry.* **128**: 379–83.

58. Willcox DL, Yovich JL, McColm SC, *et al.* (1985) Progesterone, cortisol and oestradiol 17B in the initiation of human parturition: Partitioning between free and bound hormone in plasma. *British Journal of Obstetrics and Gynaecology.* **92**: 65–71.

59. Kuevi V, Carson R, Dixon AF, *et al.* (1983) Plasma amine and hormone changes in 'postpartum blues'. *Clinical Endocrinology.* **19**: 39–46.

60. Butler J and Leonard BE. (1986) Postpartum depression and the effect of nomifensine treatment. *International Clinical Psychopharmacology.* **1**: 244–52.

61. Harris B, Fung H, McGregor A, *et al.* (1989) The hormonal environment of postnatal depression. *British Journal of Psychiatry.* **154**: 660–7.

62. Alder EM, Cook A, Davidson D, *et al.* (1986) Hormones, mood and sexuality in lactating women. *British Journal of Psychiatry.* **148**: 74–9.

63. Feksi A, Harris B, Walker RF, *et al.* (1984) Maternity 'blues' and hormone levels in saliva. *Journal of Affective Disorders.* **6**: 351–5.

64. Ballinger CB, Kay DSG, Naylor GJ, *et al.* (1982) Some biochemical findings during pregnancy and after delivery in relation to mood change. *Psychological Medicine.* **12**: 549–56.

65. Dalton K. (1985) Progesterone prophylaxis used successfully in postnatal depression. *Practitioner.* **229**: 507–8.

66. Bower WH and Altschule MD. (1956) The use of progesterone in the treatment of postpartum psychosis. *New England Journal of Medicine.* **254**: 157–60.

67. Hatotani N, Nishikubo M and Kitamaya I. (1979) Periodic psychoses in the female and the reproductive process. In: (Zichella L and Panchevi P, editors) *Psychoneuroendocrinology in reproduction*. Elsevier, Amsterdam, 55–68.

68. Potter JM, Mueller UW, Hickman PE, *et al.* (1987) Corticosteroid binding globulin in normotensive and hypertensive human pregnancy. *Clinical Science.* **72**: 725–35.

69. Railton I. (1961) The use of corticoids in postpartum depression. *Journal of the American Women's Medical Association.* **16**: 450–2.

70. Handley SL, Dunn DL, Baker JM, *et al.* (1977) Mood changes in the puerperium and plasma tryptophan and cortisol concentrations. *British Medical Journal.* **ii**: 18–22.

71. Handley SL, Dunn DL, Waldron S, *et al.* (1980) Tryptophan, cortisol and puerperal mood change. *British Journal of Psychiatry.* **136**: 498–508.

72. Okano T. (1989) Clinico-endocrine study of maternity blues. *Mie Medical Journal.* **39**: 189–200.

73. Sachar EJ, Nathan RS, Asmis G, *et al.* (1980) Neuroendocrine studies of major depressive disorder. *Acta Psychiatrica Scandinavica.* **61**(suppl.280): 201–9.

74. Amino N, Mori H, Iwatani Y, *et al.* (1982) High prevalence of transient postpartum thyrotoxicosis and hypothyroidism. *New England Journal of Medicine.* **306**: 849–52.

75. Stewart DE, Addison AM, Robinson GE, *et al.* (1988) Thyroid function in psychosis following childbirth. *American Journal of Psychiatry.* **145**: 1579–81.

76. George AJ, Copeland JRM and Wilson KCM. (1980) Serum prolactin and the postpartum blues syndrome. *British Journal of Pharmacology.* **70**: 102–3.

77. Scott AIF, Whalley LJ and Legros JJ. (1989) Treatment outcome, seizure duration and neurophysin response to ECT. *Biological Psychiatry.* **25**: 585–97.

78. Whalley LJ, Robinson ICAF and Fink G. (1982) Oxytocin and neurophysin in postpartum mania. *Lancet.* **ii**: 387–8.

79. George AJ and Wilson KCM. (1983) Beta-endorphin and puerperal psychiatric symptoms. *British Journal of Pharmacology.* **80**: 493.

80. Lindstrom LH, Nyberg F, Terenius L, *et al.* (1984) CSF and plasma B-casomorphin-like opioid peptides in postpartum psychosis. *American Journal of Psychiatry.* **141**: 1059–66.

81. Metz A, Cowen PJ, Gelder MG, *et al.* (1983) Changes in platelet alpha-adrenoceptor binding postpartum: Possible relation to maternity blues. *Lancet.* **ii**: 495–8.

82. Riley DM and Watt DC. (1985) Hypercalcaemia in the aetiology of puerperal psychosis. *Biological Psychiatry.* **20**: 479–88.

83. Garza-Trevino ES, Overall JE and Hollister LE. (1992) Verapamil versus lithium in acute mania. *American Journal of Psychiatry.* **149**: 121–2.

84. Brotman AW, Farhadi AM and Gelenberg AJ. (1986) Verapamil treatment of acute mania. *Journal of Clinical Psychiatry.* **47**: 136–8.

85. Beeley L. (1986) Drugs and breast feeding. *Clinics in Obstetrics and Gynaecology.* **13**: 247–51.

86. Barnes TRE and Katona C. (1986) Susceptibility to drug-induced hypotension in postpartum psychosis. *International Clinical Psychopharmacology.* **1**: 74–6.

87. Henderson AF, Gregoire AJP, Kumar RC, *et al.* (1991) Treatment of severe postnatal depression with oestradiol skin patches. *Lancet.* **338**: 816–7.

88. de Smit DNW and de Waart C. (1962) Relatie tussen amientiele psychose in het puerperium en het asco-binezuur-gehalte in het plasma. *Nederlands Tijdschrift voor Geneeskunde.* **106**: 159–62.

89. Daynes G. (1975) Vitamin B_{12} and puerperal psychosis. *Suid Afrikaanse Mediese Tydskrif,* 1373.

90. Lindsay JSB and Pollard DE. (1978) Mothers and children in hospital. *Australian and New Zealand Journal of Psychiatry.* **12**: 245–53.

91. Margison FR. (1990) Infants of mentally ill mothers: The risk of injury and its control. *Journal of Reproductive and Infant Psychology.* **8**: 137–46.

92. Harvey I and McGrath G. (1988) Psychiatric morbidity in spouses of women admitted to a mother and baby unit. *British Journal of Psychiatry.* **152**: 506–10.

Further Reading

Appleby L. (1990) The aetiology of postpartum psychosis: Why are there no answers? *Journal of Reproductive and Infant Psychology.* **8**: 109–18.

Deakin JFW. (1988) Relevance of hormone–CNS interactions to psychological changes in the puerperium. In: (Kumar R and Brockington IF, editors) *Motherhood and Mental Illness 2.* Wright, London, 113–32.

Hamilton JA. (1982) Model utility in postpartum psychosis. *Psychopharmacology Bulletin.* **18**: 184–7.

Hays P and Douglass A. (1984) A comparison of puerperal psychosis and the schizophreniform variant of manic-depression. *Acta Psychiatrica Scandinavica.* **69**: 177–81.

Kendell RE, Chalmers JC and Platz C. (1987) Epidemiology of puerperal psychoses. *British Journal of Psychiatry.* **159**: 662–73.

Kendell RE. (1985) Emotional and physical factors in the genesis of puerperal mental disorders. *Journal of Psychosomatic Research.* **29**: 3–11.

McGorry P and Connell S. (1990) The nosology and prognosis of puerperal psychosis. *Comprehensive Psychiatry.* **31**: 519–34.

Platz C and Kendell RE. (1988) A matched control study and family study of puerperal psychosis. *British Journal of Psychiatry.* **153**: 90–4.

Thuwe I. (1974) Genetic factors in puerperal psychosis. *British Journal of Psychiatry.* **125**: 378–85.

Wieck A. (1989) Endocrine aspects of postnatal mental disorders. *Baillière's Clinical Obstetrics and Gynaecology.* **3**: 857–77.

7 Other Relevant Psychiatric Problems

Disorders of the Mother–Baby Relationship

There is some disagreement about whether such disorders are the cause or the effect of other psychiatric illnesses of the puerperium.

Attachment has been defined as '... an enduring and unique emotional relationship between two people which is specific and endures through time'[1]. A concept which concentrates on the maternal aspect of the relationship is that of '... the extent to which the mother feels that her infant occupies an essential position in her life'[2].

Early attachment of mothers and babies has been studied by many authors by means of interview, time-lapse photography and video recording. Each of these has its own disadvantages; for example mothers may react differently when observed, or give 'acceptable' rather than true answers to interviewers. Different researchers may also have widely differing criteria of what constitutes 'attachment' or good mothering.

There are few answers to the question of what is good attachment, or how early it should appear. Using mothers' reports as a criterion, 40% of mothers in one study reported 'mainly indifference' to their newborns, 4% said that they first felt affection within 24 hours, and nearly 20% described spontaneous feeling of affection within the first three postpartum days[3]. However, the mother's mental state and events surrounding the delivery may affect their reporting of events as well as their actual behaviour.

The baby, of course has its own contribution to make to the interaction[4,5], but in terms of the mother's attitude, there appear to be two main factors to satisfactory attachment: her internal emotional response to her child, and her responsiveness to its needs. These issues can be affected by many factors, both internal and external to the mother (*see* Case Study 7.1).

Social and Cultural Factors

We have already seen that external influences such as culture, race, or religious aspects of the mother's environment may have a profound effect on her perception of the value of a child. In China, for example, where it is disapproved of to have more than one child, it is vital to the family for that child to be a boy. There is no provision for the elderly except the income from a son; a daughter becomes a member of her husband's family, and is not expected to contribute to her own parents in old age. Also, in agricultural communities, where it is important to have sons to work the land, girls are less valued. Cultural and social class factors have been clearly shown to affect mothers' behaviour in the early neonatal period[6,7].

The Experience Within the Family of Origin

Early experience such as a childhood disrupted by death or separation from either parent has been shown to be related to mothers' difficulties in managing young babies[8,9]. These mothers seemed to interact less, and to report more disturbances in the children. Clearly a woman who has had a good experience of mothering herself, or one who has also seen younger siblings cared for affectionately, will have an internal 'role model' on which to base her maternal behaviour. Alternatively, those who have been left to care for younger siblings themselves when the mother was absent, incompetent or uncaring, may associate child care with deprivation and resentment.

The relationship with the new maternal grandmother may be equally important[10], in providing both a current model for the new mother, and nurturing, praise and encouragement when she needs it most.

The Mother's Previous Experience with Babies

Anxiety in an unfamiliar situation can of course inhibit confidence and affectionate behaviour. It has been shown that multiparae are more responsive to the needs of their babies at an earlier stage than primiparae[11], and that the latter are less confident, especially when there is early separation due to a baby needing special care[12].

Primiparae experienced in child care were found to express more affection for their new babies than those without such experience[3]. Nevertheless, this previous experience may have a negative effect later in the puerperium. Women who have trained in child care, for example as paediatric nurses or nannies, may have high expectations of their responses to their own children, and be unprepared for the strong ambivalence which most mothers feel at times. They are also used to 'free time', and a financial reward for their work, neither of which may be provided when they have their own children.

The Mother's Personality

Two studies have looked at aspects of the mother's femininity or masculinity[3,13], but the results are somewhat conflicting. Perhaps more important is her predisposition to anxiety, or her dependence on others. Successful mothering depends on sensitivity to the needs of another, and confidence in making frequent and important decisions as a result of those perceptions. Those who have never had the experience of living apart from parents or spouse, those who have never had a responsible position at work, or those who have had difficulty with interpersonal relationships, may find this overwhelming.

Factors Related to Pregnancy and Delivery

The perception by the pregnant mother of the fetus as a separate person appears to have a beneficial effect on early bonding[14]. The effect of seeing the baby on a scan may reinforce this[15].

The effect of the mother's perception of the labour on her early mood state has already been discussed in Chapter three (the early puerperium). Both the difficulty of the labour and the extent of analgesic medication given to the mother may affect her responsivity[3,16,17]. Pain, discomfort and exhaustion may lead her to reject the baby at first, with subsequent guilt at her lack of 'normal' response. In one detailed study, the three most powerful factors in predicting poor early attachment were found to be artificial rupture of the membranes, painful delivery, and pethidine dosage in labour[3].

A prospective study which looked at attitudes in pregnancy, delivery, and up to six weeks postpartum found that the most significant predictors of later poor parenting were to be noted in the delivery room[18]. Perhaps observations of the parents' initial reaction should form a routine and important part of the labour record.

The Baby's Contribution to the Interaction

Clearly babies who have been exposed to large amounts of analgesic medication during labour will be less responsive and less alert at birth, hence evoking less response from the parents[17]. Neonates have been shown to have a large repertoire of response to adult communication, in terms of eye contact, imitation and vocalization; if this is impaired by drug effects, the mother's response may be harder to maintain.

Anxiety about the baby's physical state may also lead to an unconscious withholding of attachment in the early stages. Particularly with prematurity, where the baby may not conform to the mother's expectation of what a baby should look like, and where separation into a special care unit is needed, attachment will be more difficult[19] (*see* Case Study 7.2).

Visible deformities, such as angiomata, cleft lip, or Down's syndrome, may give rise to initial rejection of the child. These may lead to a period of grieving for the 'perfect' child; the time needed for full acceptance of the handicap will vary[20].

The Effect of Early Contact

Several studies have examined the effect of increased early contact between mother and baby in the later acquisition of good mothering skills and in child development. The amount of early contact has varied enormously from 15 minutes naked contact in the labour room, to continuous rooming-in. Many of these studies were carried out in 'Third World' countries with poor obstetric facilities, and in predominantly low social class subjects, so that the results may not generalize. However, overall, there are indications that increased early contact may result in more affectionate and stimulating behaviour from the mother, and that this effect may persist for some years after the birth[4,21,22]. Perhaps more importantly, mothers whose babies 'roomed-in' rated themselves as more confident and competent[23,24].

Other authors have taken the opposite path, of examining those mother–infant pairs who experienced early separation. Little difference was found at four months, and other factors such as socio-economic status and the gender of the infant appeared to be more important in the longer term[19,25].

Postpartum Stress Reaction

Several authors have recently and independently described the onset of panic disorder arising for the first time in the postnatal period[26–28]. In all cases, this seemed to originate in the woman's experience of childbirth as a dangerous or life-threatening event, in spite of a satisfactory outcome for mother and child.

Although anxiety symptoms have been associated with depression, these women did not appear to describe typical depressive symptoms, and they had no prior history of depression or panic disorder, although there was a positive family history of panic disorder in a few of the reported cases[28].

The panic attacks appear to be typical, consisting of a feeling of dread associated with trembling, palpitations, a feeling of tightness in the chest or neck, overbreathing, and a 'churning' stomach. These women feel at worst that they might die in the attack, or at least that they might collapse or vomit.

The incidence is usually worse when out of the house, and may lead to a secondary agoraphobia. Even at home, there are real worries about being left alone with the baby when at such times they are incapable of caring for it.

The onset is typically either during, or immediately following, the delivery, and there is sometimes a partial amnesia for the birth itself. The onset of amnesia coincides with the occurrence of dissociative symptoms. A typical case history is reported as follows:

A 28-year-old woman complained of emotional numbing, sleep disturbances, anxiety and intrusive thoughts
since the birth of her twins two years before. She had
a long history of infertility and had been confined to
bed for the last months of her pregnancy because of
hydramnios. During this time, she had recurrent
thoughts that her abdomen would rupture and she
would lose her twins. When labour started, she developed a panic reaction which ceased when she felt as if
she had left her body and 'hovered' over her abdomen
'like a ghost'. Back on the ward, she was restless and
complained of frightening intrusive memories of the
delivery. She denied any previous symptoms of panic,
anxiety or dissociation until this delivery[28].

Thus the symptoms appear to originate in extreme anxiety
regarding the delivery, often in women with 'overvalued' pregnancies, for example, those following a period of infertility, or
previous miscarriages. They fear a disastrous result to the
current pregnancy, and their anxiety results in dissociative
symptoms at the time, with repetitive and distressing thoughts
and memories at a later date. The syndrome can occur even
when the pregnancy is not especially precious, but where the
delivery is experienced as potentially life-threatening for either
mother or child.

These women seem to lose faith in the safety of the outside
world, seeing danger in all situations, and even losing faith in
the integrity of their own bodies. They may become hypochondriacal, or over-anxious about the baby's health. Because of this
exaggerated anxiety they feel unable to let others care for the
child (*see* Case Study 7.3).

The lack of attachment to the baby reported by many women
seems to be part of a general emotional numbness. Where this
extends to the partner, it may lead to relationship and sexual
problems[26], especially since a further pregnancy is contemplated with the utmost fear.

Further medical contact is often avoided, since it revives
painful memories, so that many of these women do not present
for help until much later.

Post-traumatic stress disorder is defined as:

- the experience of an event which is outside the range of usual experience and which would be markedly distressing to almost anyone

- the traumatic event is persistently re-experienced in at least one of the following ways:
  - recurrent and distressing recollections of the trauma
  - recurrent and distressing dreams of the trauma
  - suddenly acting or feeing as if the trauma had recurred
  - intense psychological distress at exposure to events that symbolize or resemble the trauma

- persistent avoidance of stimuli associated with the trauma as indicated by at least three of the following:
  - efforts to avoid thoughts of the trauma
  - efforts to avoid activities or situations that arouse memories of the trauma
  - inability to recall important aspects of the trauma
  - markedly diminished interest in significant activities
  - feeling of detachment from others
  - restricted range of affect (eg emotional numbing)

- persistent symptoms of increased arousal as evidenced by at least two of the following:
  - difficulty falling or staying asleep
  - irritability or outbursts of anger
  - difficulty concentrating
  - hypervigilance
  - exaggerated startle response
  - physiological reactivity on exposure to events that symbolize or resemble an aspect of the trauma.

It could be argued that childbirth is not an event that is outside the range of usual experience, although it is certainly possible that some of these complicated deliveries would be 'markedly distressing to almost anyone'. We also know that life-threatening events actually do occur in 0.19% of all deliveries[29]. Nevertheless, in these women it is their subjective experience that is important. What, after all, could be worse than the fear of losing the long-awaited baby, or of losing one's own life in giving birth? In all other respects, they conform to the above diagnostic criteria.

This syndrome has been called the 'partus stress reaction'[28], and, in clinical experience, occurs in approximately 2/1000 deliveries, although those referred for psychiatric care may be only a small fraction of the total number. Those most susceptible would appear to be women with a past personal or family history of panic disorder, those with a particular need for control, and those sensitive to 'loss of status' at giving up a career.

There is some evidence that pre-existing panic disorder partially remits during pregnancy, and it is possible that the postpartum exacerbation is a rebound phenomenon. It has been postulated that the improvement in pregnancy is related to high progesterone levels[30], or that the puerperal exacerbation is due to changes in α-2-adrenergic receptor function[27].

Treatment

Recognition of the condition is the first requirement. It should be clearly distinguished from postnatal depression on the basis of the presenting symptoms and the time of onset in relation to the delivery.

The woman's own experience rather than the technical details of the birth should be validated, not minimized or contradicted. She will need continued opportunities to recount the events and her accompanying feelings. Writing a full account of the traumatic events can also be therapeutic. Explanation of the symptoms is helpful, so that she herself can make sense of her experience, and not feel, as so many do, that she is 'going mad'.

In the presence of such marked anxiety, it is unlikely that these women can make use of relaxation techniques, but simple self-help instructions are reassuring (*see* Appendix 7.1). Formal relaxation training may be helpful at a later stage of the illness, but will need repeated daily practice to be effective. Suitable relaxation audiotapes are available from most chain store chemists and stationers.

Beta-blockers such as propranolol can reduce the physical accompaniments of panic, allowing the mother to undertake normal activities, and to build up her confidence. They have the additional advantage of being non-sedating.

Where secondary depressive symptoms are present, monoamine oxidase inhibitors such as phenelzine or tranylcypromine are helpful, although contra-indicated in breast-feeding mothers. Tricyclic antidepressants are not usually effective, and the side-effects may add to the anxiety about physical problems.

Benzodiazepines are best avoided because of the potential for escalating the dose and for addiction.

Pregnancy and Childbirth in Survivors of Childhood Sexual Abuse

Little has been written on this subject, which is nevertheless an important issue in maternity care. We know that the prevalence of childhood sexual abuse is high. Approximately 40% of women in community surveys report some sexual approach in their childhood, and over 20% report actual physical contact[31,32]. The prevalence in women presenting with psychiatric problems is even higher.

Late Effects

There are many late effects of childhood sexual abuse, including:

Low self-esteem
These women feel guilty, ashamed, and blame themselves, not only for the abuse, but for everything that goes wrong in their lives[33,34]. As children they felt 'different' as a result of their experience, which they feel is exclusive to themselves. This can result in poor relationships within their peer group, and a lifelong difficulty with interpersonal relationships (*see* Case Study 7.4).

Depression
There is an overwhelming feeling of helplessness and hopelessness, with an extremely negative view of their own self-worth[35]. If we adopt Seligman's[36] view of the origins of depression, it is not surprising that many of these women are chronically depressed.

Sadness and grief may also be a bereavement reaction for the caring parents she never had, or the childhood that came to a premature end (*see* Case Study 7.5).

Chaotic life-style

'Victim' behaviour may persist into adult life[37], and reproduce itself in terms of masochistic relationships or addictions to drugs or alcohol. The latter also have the effect of 'blotting out' the traumatic memories.

Survivors may leave home prematurely to escape the abuse, making them more vulnerable to further exploitation. Even early marriages often fail because of problems with intimacy, trust and sexuality. The divorce and separation rate is higher in these women[37].

Sexual problems

Many of these women have an aversion to physical contact, and sexual problems are almost the norm. Any sexual activity may lead to 'flashbacks' to her childhood experience and intense anxiety. Sexual arousal may be impaired or absent, often due to dissociation from sexual feelings. They often describe feeling 'numb' in the genital area. Intense feelings of guilt may arise at orgasm if this was experienced during the early abuse[38].

Anger

Some survivors show extreme anger and rage towards the world in general and to family and friends in particular[39]. They may not associate this with justifiable rage towards the abuser, nor may the recipients understand the cause. This further alienates them from support and reinforces feelings of unworthiness.

Emotional numbing

The child's defence to the trauma is to cut herself off from emotional response, sometimes to the point of dissociation[34]. This inability to accept feelings may lead to somatic symptoms, and this is contributed to by the real fear of having been damaged by the abuse.

Confusion

Mental confusion is a prominent feature in many ex-victims[38]. This may arise from the attempt to make sense of sexual knowledge in childhood, or from ambivalence to the abuser. The survivor is therefore unable to make judgements about other people, or indeed, herself. This is also a reason for poor scholastic achievement and lack of qualifications, and hence a further lack of self-worth[40].

Need for control

Having felt that their early lives were under the control of others, some women compensate by controlling their adult lives in a maladaptive way. Obsessive–compulsive disorder is common, especially in relation to cleaning rituals, which may also have a symbolic meaning in cleansing themselves from the abuse[41].

Anorexia may represent not only control, but a denial of sexuality, and the secret bingeing and vomiting of bulimia may re-enact the shame and disgust associated with the abuse[42]. Compulsive eating is often part of a survivor's difficulty with control, and being overweight has the added advantage of making her less desirable so that sexual activity can be avoided.

Self-harm

Self-mutilation occurs in the more disturbed women. The motivation may be punishment, distraction from intrusive memories, or a need to reassure herself that she can still perceive pain. Suicide attempts occur when the memories become too powerful, or when her control over her current life experience becomes too difficult[37].

Anxiety

This is common in survivors, either as free-floating anxiety and panic disorder, or specific fears and phobias which relate to the circumstances of the abuse. Fear of hospitals and medical procedures is common. In such cases, hospital represents a loss of identity and control, a lack of privacy, and a feeling of being trapped.

Implications During Pregnancy

Becoming a parent for the first time is a powerful trigger for the re-awakening of these past traumatic experiences. After all, pregnancy is an advertisement to the world at large that the survivor has engaged in sexual activity, and this, in itself, may be a cause for shame and guilt.

There is also the need to attend clinics, and to be examined internally, repeating the physical position and feelings of help-lessness in the presence of authority figures, leading to 'flash-backs' to the abuse. She may feel damaged internally from her previous experience, and be afraid that this will be discovered by those examining her. She may also fear that her child may be abnormal in some way, either as a result of the abuse, or as a 'punishment'. Some therapists have even postulated that she may have fantasies about the child being the abuser's, not her partner's.

Implications Postpartum

The survivor may be able to feel good about herself during pregnancy, especially as a result of extra attention, and the feeling that she is creating a new, innocent, unspoiled child. However, after the birth, she may feel that only the baby is good, and that she reverts to being 'bad' – not good enough to be a mother – and these feelings lead to self-hate and depression.

There is also the anxiety about whether she will be able to protect her child from similar abuse. These mothers often become over-protective, unable to leave the baby in the care of others, especially the partner, and hence feel 'trapped' and confined. This anxiety seems to be more common with female children, whilst with boys, there may be fear and rejection of their developing masculine traits. This can certainly be a problem with lively and aggressive toddlers.

The lack of proper parenting in her own childhood may leave her poorly equipped to deal with the demands of caring for her own children. She may even fear becoming a perpetrator herself, as mothers are generally aware that there is a high incidence of child abuse amongst those abused themselves in childhood.

She may have seen her own mother as collusive or weak, and will undoubtedly have felt intense anger towards her. This prevents her accepting practical or emotional support from her family, especially if the abuser is still living in the parental home.

The Professional's Role

It is sometimes difficult for professional carers to believe that the problem is so widespread, and the initial tendency is to wish to deny that it exists.

Most women will not disclose the abuse, which may be detected by their attitudes to medical procedures. They may be irregular attenders at antenatal clinics, although most will want to attend for reassurance that all is well. Midwives may detect undue embarrassment at being examined, or excessive concern about the normality of the pregnancy. There may for example, be specific phobias about venepuncture.

Many survivors wish to control the circumstances of delivery, asking for a home confinement, or presenting a detailed birth plan. They may refuse analgesia in labour because they fear loss of control, and may be angry and resentful if intervention is needed. Problems with trust in authority figures may lead the mother to question the competence of those caring for her. Because of antipathy to physical closeness, she may handle the baby ineptly, or refuse to breast-feed. There may be an insistence on early discharge from hospital.

If the underlying reason for this behaviour is not understood, these women may be seen as 'difficult', and arouse resentment in the staff.

Postnatally, depression is common. If the health visitor or family doctor are involved in counselling and support, and make a good relationship with the mother, she may feel sufficiently confident to disclose the earlier abuse. The way in which this is received will be all-important. Professionals are sometimes reluctant to accept this information. They may feel that they lack both expertize and time to deal with it, and may fear 'doing more harm than good' by becoming involved.

Accepting and validating the woman's experience can never be harmful. Most women have reached adulthood with their own defence mechanisms in place, and many will be ambivalent or reluctant to embark on formal therapy. In most cases, empathy and sensitivity from professional carers will allow the mother to explore her anxieties in a safe setting. It is most important that disclosures made in confidence should be kept absolutely confidential. This information should not be passed on to colleagues without the mother's express permission, and should not be recorded in the notes except in coded form.

Reassurance and encouragement of her mothering skills will be needed. She may be ultra-sensitive to rejection, and it is important to keep appointments punctually, and to give her full attention during the consultation. A referral for more specialized counselling should be made if she expresses a wish for it. Persuading her to accept it will be self-defeating.

Case Study 7.1

Marion was a 33-year-old woman referred by her family doctor three months after the birth of her first child. The pregnancy had been unplanned, and she described feeling 'devastated' when it was confirmed. She had had two episodes of bleeding early in the pregnancy, and had hoped that she would miscarry. She detached herself emotionally from the pregnancy throughout, and her husband appeared to do the same. She continued to work full-time until 38 weeks.

Labour was quick and normal, and the baby was healthy. She felt 'disbelief' on seeing the child and did not want to touch or to hold him. The husband said that his only feeling was of being 'overwhelmed' at being burdened with a child 'for the next 18 years'.

For the first two weeks after the birth she felt somewhat elated in mood, but, on her husband's return to work, felt miserable, abandoned and irritable. She admitted that were it not for public opinion and the feelings of her own mother, she would gladly offer the baby for adoption. She regarded it as a duty to look after him, and did so mechanically, with no feelings of affection or tenderness. The child seemed discontented and unhappy, with no eye contact and poor social responses.

A family aide was helpful in encouraging her undoubted competence in the physical care of the baby, and acting as a role model for play activities with him. Marion did not do well in a self-help group for mothers as she felt her problems were quite different from those of the other group members. However, she benefited from some individual counselling sessions. She then found a suitable child-minder and returned to part-time work. Following this her relationship with her son improved.

She still feels angry with her husband who has made no effort to adjust to fatherhood. The future of the marriage is currently in doubt.

Case Study 7.2

Mary was a 29-year-old woman who presented five months after the delivery of her second child. The pregnancy had been unplanned and unwelcome, but she had not contemplated termination. The baby, a boy, was born at 34 weeks' gestation, and spent two weeks in special care. On his return home, she found that she had no affection for him, could not tolerate his crying, and, at times, felt that she wanted to harm him. She had been unable to care for him at all during the previous six weeks.

Mary's childhood had been very unhappy. Her father was an alcoholic and violent to his wife and three children, sexually abusing Mary from the age of four years. Her mother had been aware of the abuse, but had been powerless to stop it.

During Mary's first marriage she had two late miscarriages due to genetic defects. Her second marriage was happy, and she had a two-year-old daughter whom she adored. However, she had extreme anxiety about possible abuse of her daughter, always dressing her like a boy to 'protect' her. She spontaneously related some of her feelings about her son to anger with her father.

She was admitted to the mother and baby unit for assessment of her mental state, and of her bonding to her son. There was no evidence of depression. Her feelings towards the baby improved remarkably and quite quickly, and she was discharged with a full programme of community support, having already embarked on a series of counselling sessions addressing her history of sexual abuse.

A few months later, she was pregnant again, and, after the birth of a second daughter, again rejected her son. Persistent attempts to rehabilitate the family failed, and she finally insisted, against her husband's wishes, that the child should be offered for adoption.

Mary's husband is now receiving counselling for his depressive reaction to separation from his son.

Case Study 7.3

Anita was referred two years after the birth of her first child when she was 40 years old. She had been a senior management consultant involved in university teaching and research. Her husband was 58 with two grown and married children. They had recently moved house and area and had no close friends.

The pregnancy was planned and normal, and she worked until 39 weeks. Induction was performed at 41 weeks for mild hypertension and postmaturity. Breech presentation was diagnosed, and she was advised to have a caesarian section. However, a second examination revealed a cephalic presentation and she had a trial of labour with an attempted forceps delivery, followed by a caesarian section under general anaesthesia. The puerperium was complicated by a pelvic infection, and breast-feeding failed.

From the time of delivery she felt cheated and angry. She blamed the medical staff for misdiagnosing the presentation, and the nursing staff for feeding the baby and causing breast-feeding problems.

She had flashbacks to the time of delivery, and sometimes woke in the night convinced that she was still in the labour ward. Her major complaints were of 'confusion', poor concentration, and loss of confidence. She found it impossible to think logically, and felt that her career was at an end.

She was extremely anxious about her own health, pursuing many different medical opinions for gynaecological and physical problems, and had not been able to work since the birth. She was also extremely anxious about the baby's health, and unable to leave her in the care of others.

Individual counselling sessions helped her to see that she had experienced a traumatic event, but was not irreparably damaged as she had feared. She was able to take on some consultant work from home and her confidence returned.

Case Study 7.4

Serena was referred when she was 25 weeks into a second planned pregnancy. She suffered from severe nausea and vomiting in the early stages, and complained of labile mood for the previous three months. She had been miserable, anxious, panicky, and jealous of her husband to the point where she could not bear him to watch television in case attractive women were on the screen.

She had also been dieting, restricting her intake to toast and soup once daily, and abusing laxatives if she ate more than this.

Serena's father had been a distant, frightening man who drank heavily and had been violent to his wife. There was also a younger sister who had taken frequent overdoses and had self-mutilated since her teens.

Her first marriage was to an alcoholic and a gambler. Her one pregnancy from this marriage ended in a miscarriage at 20 weeks, and the relationship ended after three years. Her present husband was kind and affectionate. There were no housing or financial problems.

Serena and her sister had been sexually abused by their father over a prolonged period of time. She had married young to escape from the abuse, and felt that she had been 'punished' by the loss of her first child. She felt that she did not 'deserve' her present happy relationship, and that further disasters such as the loss of this baby or of her husband, were inevitable.

She was able to see the connection between her fears and her low self-esteem. She confided in her husband, who was supportive, but she did not feel that she wished for any further counselling at the time.

Case Study 7.5

Ruth, a 34-year-old woman, presented when 20 weeks into her second pregnancy, with depression, irritability and sleep disturbance. She was happily married, comfortably housed and had a two-year-old daughter. The current pregnancy was planned.

She became very tearful when talking about her family of origin. It emerged that she had been sexually abused by her father for several years from the age of 10. She had successfully suppressed the knowledge of the abuse until she saw a television programme on the subject, when '... the memories came flooding back'.

In some distress, she telephoned a national helpline. During a prolonged conversation with the counsellor, she was persuaded that confrontation of her father was essential. This she duly did, with disastrous consequences. Her mother was horrified, and immediately left her own home to live with Ruth, being distressed and angry with her daughter for the breakup of her marriage. Ruth also felt that her mother blamed her for the original abuse.

It was arranged that she should have some individual counselling sessions during the remainder of her pregnancy. After the birth, she participated in time-limited group therapy with other survivors. She began to appreciate that she was responsible neither for the abuse nor her mother's distress. She was able to see that she had been able to make close relationships and was a good mother to her children in spite of her traumatic experience.

Appendix 7.1

INSTRUCTION CHART FOR PANIC ATTACKS

- Remember that the feelings are no more than an exaggeration of the normal bodily reactions to stress.

- They are not in the least harmful or dangerous – just unpleasant. Nothing worse will happen.

- Stop adding to panic with frightening thoughts about what is happening and where it might lead.

- Describe to yourself what is really happening in your body at this moment, not what you fear may happen.

- Now wait and give the fear time to pass without fighting it or running away from it. Just accept it.

- Notice that one you stop adding to it with frightening thoughts, the fear starts to fade away by itself.

- Remember that the whole point of practice is learning how to cope with fear without avoiding it, so this is an opportunity to make progress.

- Think about the progress you have made so far despite all the difficulties, and how pleased you will be when you succeed this time.

- Now begin to describe your surroundings to yourself, and plan out in your mind exactly what to do next.

- Then, when you are ready to go, start off in an easy, relaxed way. There is no need for effort or hurry.

References

1. Kennell JH, Voos DK and Klaus MH. (1979) Parent–infant bonding. In: (Osofsky J, editor.) *Handbook of infant development*. Wiley, Chichester, 786–8.

2. Robson KS and Moss HA. (1970) Patterns and determinants of maternal attachment. *Journal of Pediatrics*. **77**: 976–85.

3. Robson KM and Kumar R. (1980) Delayed onset of maternal affection after childbirth. *British Journal of Psychiatry*. **136**: 347–53.

4. de Chateau P and Wiberg B. (1977) Long-term effect on mother–infant behaviour of extra contact during the first hour postpartum: 1. *Acta Paediatrica Scandinavica*. **66**: 137–43.

5. Stern D. (1977) *The first relationship: Infant and Mother*. Fontana, London.

6. Klaus MH, Trouse MA and Kennell JH. (1975) Does human maternal behaviour after delivery show a characteristic pattern? In: Porter E and O'Connor M, *CIBA Foundation Symposium 33: Parent –infant interaction*. Elsevier, Excerpta Medica, North Holland, 69–85.

7. Dunn JF. Understanding human development: Limitations and possibilities in an ethological approach. In: (von Cranach M, editor.) *Human ethology*. Cambridge University Press, Cambridge, 623–62.

8. Frommer EA and O'Shea G. (1973) Antenatal identification of women liable to have problems managing their infants. *British Journal of Psychiatry*. **123**: 149–56.

9. Hall F, Pawlby SJ and Wolkind S. (1980) Early life experiences and later mothering behaviour. In: (Schaffer D and Dunn J, editors.) *The first year of life: Psychological and medical implications of early experience*. Wiley, Chichester, 153–74.

10. Uddenberg N. (1974) Reproductive adaptation in mother and daughter. *Acta Psychiatrica Scandinavica*. Suppl 254.

11. Bernal J. (1972) Crying during the first 10 days of life and maternal responses. *Developmental Medicine and Child Neurology*. **14**: 362.

12. Seashore MJ, Leifer AD, Barnett R, *et al.* (1973) The effects of denial of early mother–infant interaction on maternal self-confidence. *Journal of Personality and Social Psychology*. **26**: 369–78.

13. Breen D. (1975) *The birth of a first child*. Tavistock, London.

14. Bibring GL, Dwyer TF, Huntington DS, *et al.* (1961) A study of psychological processes in pregnancy of the earliest mother–child relationship: 1. *Psychoanalytic Study of the Child*. **16**: 9–27.

15. Campbell S, Reading AE, Cox DN, *et al.* (1982) Ultrasound scanning in pregnancy: The short term psychological effects of early real-time scans. *Journal of Psychosomatic Obstetrics and Gynaecology*. **1**: 57–61.

16. Brown NJV, Bakeman R, Snyder PA, *et al.* (1975) The interactions of black inner-city mothers with their newborn infants. *Child Development*. **46**: 677–86.

17. Rosenblatt D, Redshaw M, Packer M, *et al.* (1979) Drugs, birth and infant behaviour. *New Scientist*. **83**: 487–9.

18. Ball JA. (1987) *Reactions to motherhood*. Cambridge University Press, Cambridge.

19. Leifer GD, Leiderman PH, Barnett CR, *et al.* (1972) Effects of mother–infant separation on maternal attachment behaviour. *Child Development*. **43**: 1203–18.

20. Nippert I. (1990) Coping with severe birth defects – a report from a 4-year longitudinal study. *Journal of Psychosomatic Obstetrics and Gynaecology*. **11** (Special Issue 1): 83–90.

21. Newton N and Newton M. (1962) Mothers' reactions to their newborn babies. *JAMA*. **181**: 206–10.

22. Hales DJ, Lozoff B, Sosa R, *et al.* (1977) Defining the limits of the maternal sensitive period. *Developmental Medicine and Child Neurology*. **19**: 454–561.

23. Greenberg M. (1973) First mothers rooming-in with their newborns: Its impact on the mother. *American Journal of Orthopsychiatry*. **43**: 783–8.

24. O'Connor S, Vietze PM, Sherrod KB, *et al.* (1980) Reduced incidence of parenting inadequacy following rooming-in. *Pediatrics.* **66**: 176–82.

25. Leiderman PH and Seashore MJ. (1975) Mother–infant separation: Some delayed consequences. In: Porter E and O'Connor M, *CIBA Foundation Symposium 33: Parent–infant Interaction.* Elsevier, Excerpta Medica, North Holland. 213–32.

26. Bloor RN and Jones RA. (1988) Post-traumatic stress disorder and sexual dysfunction. *British Journal of Sexual Medicine.* **15**: 170–2.

27. Metz A, Sichel DA and Goff DC. (1988) Postpartum panic disorder. *Journal of Clinical Psychiatry.* **49**: 278–9.

28. Moleman N, van der Hart O and van der Kolk BA. (1992) The partus stress reaction: A neglected aetiological factor in postpartum psychiatric disorders. *Journal of Nervous and Mental Disease.* **180**: 271–2.

29. Stones W, Lim W, Al-Azzawi F, *et al.* (1991) An investigation of maternal morbidity with identification of life-threatening 'near-miss' episodes. *Health Trends* **23**: 13–15.

30. Villeponteaux VA, Lydiard RB, Laraia MT, *et al.* (1992) The effects of pregnancy on pre-existing panic disorder. *Journal of Clinical Psychiatry.* **53**: 201–3.

31. West DJ, editor. (1985) *Sexual Victimisation.* Aldershot, Gower.

32. Baker AW and Duncan SP. (1985) Child sexual abuse: A study of prevalence in Great Britain. *Child Abuse and Neglect.* **9**: 457–67.

33. Kempe RS and Kempe CH. (1984) *The Common Secret: Sexual Abuse of Children and Adolescents.* Freeman, New York.

34. Hall L and Lloyd S. (1989) *Surviving Child Sexual Abuse.* Falmer Press, New York.

35. Browne A and Finkelhor D. (1986) *A Sourcebook of Child Sexual Abuse.* Sage, Beverly Hill, 143–79.

36. Seligman MEP. (1985) *Helplessness: On depression, development and death.* WH Freeman, San Francisco.

37. Russell DEH. (1986) *The Secret Trauma: Incest in the Lives of Girls and Women.* Basic Books, New York.

38. Gelinas D. (1983) The persisting negative effects of incest. *Psychiatry.* **46**: 312–22.

39. Hays KF. (1985) Electra in mourning: Grief work and the adult incest survivor. *Psychotherapy Patient.* **2**: 45–58.

40. Nakashima I and Zakus G. (1977) Incest review and clinical experience. *Pediatrics.* **60**: 696–701.

41. Winestine MC. (1985) Compulsive shoplifting as a derivative of childhood seduction. *Psychoanalytic Quarterly.* **54**: 70–2.

42. Sloan G and Leichner P. (1986) Is there a relationship between sexual abuse or incest and eating disorders? *Canadian Journal of Psychiatry.* **31**: 656–70.

8   Psychotropic Drugs

Psychotropic Drugs in Pregnancy

Women are currently bombarded with advice about what is harmful to the fetus. They know that smoking and alcohol can affect the development of the baby, and they take care to have a healthy and balanced diet, avoiding foods such as soft cheeses which may carry a risk of intrauterine infection. They are therefore naturally reluctant to take any kind of medication during pregnancy, and rightly so.

However, not all pregnancies are planned, and some may occur when the mother is already taking medication. Alternatively, the hazards of not accepting treatment may be so severe, that the risk may be considered to be justifiable in an individual case. In either of these scenarios, the mother and her advisors need accurate and easily accessible information about any possible ill effects of the drug on the fetus in order to make an informed decision about whether the pregnancy should continue.

Medication can affect the fetus in a variety of ways. The drug may be mutagenic, affecting the genetic material in the ovum even before fertilization. It may be teratogenic like thalidomide, affecting the differentiation of cells, and the development of limbs and organs. Later in pregnancy, it may increase the risk of miscarriage or impair fetal growth. Later still, it may increase the risk of prematurity or fetal death. Even after delivery, there may be direct toxic or withdrawal symptoms in the neonate. Lastly, there may be remote effects some years later. An example of this is the occurrence of vaginal carcinoma in the daughters of women given synthetic oestrogen during pregnancy up to 20 years earlier.

Fortunately for the psychiatric health of mothers, few of these adverse effects are attributable to psychotropic drugs. Nevertheless, these factors must be carefully considered for each drug used, and the risks weighed against the benefits of treatment.

For example, although suicide in pregnancy is rare, it does occur. Manic overactivity may lead to dehydration and exhaustion with adverse effects on the pregnancy. Even a mother who is severely anxious, depressed or obsessional during pregnancy may be unable to care for her existing children, with consequent disruption to the whole family. All of these situations could perhaps be prevented by cautious and informed prescribing.

Factors Affecting Risk to the Fetus

Maternal physiology

Normal changes in maternal physiology during pregnancy may affect maternal absorption, detoxification and excretion of drugs of any kind. For example, gastric emptying may be slower, hence drugs are absorbed more slowly, but possibly in higher concentrations. Plasma volume is increased, resulting in a lower serum concentration of the drug. At the same time, plasma albumin decreases, thus lowering the protein bound fraction of the medication, whilst the free fraction rises. Glomerular filtration rate and hormonally induced liver enzymes increase, leading to increased rates of metabolism and excretion.

Fetal physiology

In comparison with the adult, the blood supply to the brain and the blood–brain permeability is higher in the fetus, leading to more complete exposure of the fetal brain to maternal drugs. The fetal liver has a lower concentration of microsomal enzymes which metabolize drugs, so that the effects may be increased or prolonged. The excretion of most drugs via the placenta or fetal urine may be delayed, hence accumulation may occur.

Timing of drug administration

There appears to be no direct effect of psychotropic drugs on fertility, but haploid cells and minor chromosomal abnormalities have been reported with thioridazine and lithium. However, there is no evidence for psychotropic drugs causing an increased incidence of spontaneous abortion, which might be predicted if the chromosomal abnormalities were severe.

The greatest risk of teratogenesis is within the first 10 weeks of pregnancy. Effects on the development of the nervous system are greatest between the 10th and 25th day, on the cardiovascular system between the 20th and 40th day, and on limb development from the 24th to the 26th day.

Drugs such as opiates and benzodiazepines, which may have significant withdrawal effects, will adversely affect the fetus if given near to the time of delivery.

Neuroleptic Drugs

One of the earliest reports is of a woman treated with high doses of neuroleptic drugs throughout pregnancy: up to 400 mg of chlorpromazine or 1600 mg thioridazine daily. At 24 hours of age the baby showed extrapyramidal symptoms in the form of increased muscle tone and abnormal movements. There was improvement by seven months, and there was no developmental delay at 22 or 32 months[1]. A second child of the same mother had similar but milder symptoms after lower doses during pregnancy. Two similar cases were reported by other authors in 1969 and 1970[2,3].

Oral or intramuscular flupenthixol administered to five mothers up to the time of delivery led to cord blood concentrations of the drug of 25% of that in the maternal serum[4]. No adverse effects were noted in any of the children.

Another mother, on 200 mg fluphenazine decanoate every three weeks, had a healthy baby at 41 weeks. There were mild extrapyramidal symptoms in the infant at four weeks, but he was thriving and healthy at two months and at two years of age[5].

Several large scale studies have been carried out with somewhat contradictory results. A French survey showed that the incidence of non-chromosomal abnormalities in 315 women taking phenothiazines in the first trimester was 3.5% compared with 1.6% in a control group[6]. A report on 1309 cases of infants exposed to phenothiazines *in utero* showed no increase in congenital abnormality[7], but when the results were analysed according to the timing of the exposure, the incidence was 5.4% compared with 3.2% in controls[8]. The time of maximum risk was between six and 10 weeks into the pregnancy.

These results must be compared with the outcome of pregnancy in untreated psychotic patients who seem to have a higher risk of neonatal mortality and morbidity, independent of medication[9,10].

In a survey of 94 women taking small doses 1.2 mg/day) of haloperidol in the first trimester there were no birth defects[11]. There appears to be no increase in congenital abnormalities in women taking trifluoperazine[12,13], thioridazine or fluphenazine[14,15].

There is a single report of two cases in which the infant developed intestinal obstruction in the neonatal period[3]. This is possibly related to the anticholinergic effects of these drugs.

Long-term follow-up is reassuring: 52 children born to mothers who had taken chlorpromazine during pregnancy were said to have developed normally up to five years postpartum[16-18], and there were no differences in IQ scores at four years between 151 children exposed to phenothiazines *in utero* and a control group[7].

In view of the large number of women maintained on neuroleptic drugs over a period of many years, and the notable absence of reports of fetal abnormality, it must be concluded that there is no convincing evidence for the teratogenicity of this group of drugs. This has been confirmed in animal studies[19]. The risk of untreated psychotic illness has to be evaluated in each individual; in many cases it will outweigh the risk of medication. If the pregnancy is diagnosed early, it might be wise to omit or reduce the dosage between the sixth and 10th week. Depot medication can reduce the peaks of serum concentration; this is probably the safest route to use in pregnancy. If the mother is on medication at delivery, the paediatrician should be alerted in case of Parkinsonian or withdrawal effects in the neonate.

Antidepressants

There have been two early reports of possible teratogenic effects as a result of tricyclic administration to the mother[20,21]. Three infants had limb reduction deformities, and one anencephaly. As a result of this alarm, large scale studies have been carried out and have failed to find any association. There have been surveys of 10 000 pregnancies in England and Wales[22], 15 000 in Scotland[23], and nearly 3000 in Finland[24]. No link was found in these surveys between fetal deformities and tricyclics in pregnancy.

Some authors have reported adverse effects on the neonate

when tricyclics are administered late in pregnancy. The effects are reported to include tachycardia, irritability, tremor, and retention of urine (Geigy Pharmaceuticals and others, personal communication)[25,26]. These symptoms relate to the anticholinergic effect of the medication. Two mothers who took clomipramine (Anafranil) in doses of 100 mg and 200 mg daily had babies who were 'jittery', tachypneoic and cyanosed. Feeding difficulties persisted for 16 days in one case, but both children subsequently showed normal development[27].

Phenelzine (Nardil) has teratogenic and neurochemical effects on the young in animal studies, together with later neurobehavioural effects[28-30]. There is no information on the other MAOI antidepressants.

During the early trials with paroxetine (Seroxat), ten women became pregnant whilst taking the drug. One miscarried, four opted for termination and the remaining five had full term normal deliveries with no congenital abnormalities (Smith, Kline, Beecham, personal communication, 1994). In animal studies, no evidence of teratogenesis was found in rabbits, but a reduced pregnancy rate and increased early pregnancy wastage were found in rats[31].

A prospective study of 128 women on therapeutic doses of fluoxetine (Prozac) during the first trimester showed that there was no increase in the rate of congenital malformations in comparison with one group on tricyclic antidepressants and another on no medication[32]. The rate did not exceed that expected in the population at large, but there was a small increase in the miscarriage rate in the two treated groups (13.5% on paroxetine, 12.2% on tricyclics, and 6.8% in the untreated group).

Prescription event monitoring of fluvoxamine (Faverin) showed that 17 pregnant women were exposed to the drug during the first trimester. There were five spontaneous abortions and one ectopic pregnancy, and four women opted for termination; seven live births resulted, including one pair of twins, with no abnormalities in the infants[33].

It would appear that there is a slightly increased risk of early fetal loss associated with the use of antidepressants of any kind. Since the selective serotonin re-uptake inhibitors have been used over a relatively short period of time, they are best avoided until further information is available. The tricyclics appear to be safe, but the lowest possible dose should be used. It is also preferable to lower the dose before delivery in order to avoid withdrawal effects in the baby.

Hypnotics and Sedatives

There are reports that the maternal use of diazepam (Valium) is associated with an increased risk of oral cleft defects in the children[34-36]. In addition, a large study of 104 000 women showed that the 80 women receiving benzodiazepines during pregnancy had a rate of neurological congenital abnormalities of 13% compared with 7% in the remainder[37]. However, many of these women also abused alcohol and other illicit drugs, and had a higher incidence of pregnancy complications.

Reports on chlordiazepoxide (Librium) are contradictory. A 1974 study showed that the rates of severe congenital abnormality associated with this drug in early pregnancy were 11.4% compared with 2.4% in controls[38]. Two later large studies did not show any ill effects[22,39].

Retrospective studies have looked at women whose children were born with abnormalities, and examined their drug consumption during pregnancy. One study of 836 such women showed that the only significant association was with the use of a hormonal pregnancy test[40]. No correlation was found with benzodiazepine use, although the numbers on the drug were small.

A similar study examined the psychotropic drug use of 73 mothers whose babies suffered a perinatal death[41]. Maternal blood samples taken in early pregnancy were tested for benzodiazepines, and approximately 6–7% were found to be positive, a similar proportion to that in the control group. There was an association of benzodiazepines with impaired fetal growth and low birth weight. The cause of perinatal death in the babies exposed to benzodiazepines was malformation (including two cases of renal abnormality) in three, anoxia in three, the remaining three were unexplained.

Later in pregnancy, the effects may also be serious. High doses of diazepam given in labour have been shown to produce neonatal hypotonia, hypothermia and feeding problems[42].

Short-term use of lower doses seems to have little adverse effect[43], but, if the mother is given the drug over a long period antenatally, the effects in the baby may last for up to two weeks[44]. A withdrawal syndrome in the neonate, consisting of tremor, irritability and increased muscle tone has also been recorded[45,46].

The use of these drugs is rarely unavoidable, and, in view of their proven ill effects both early and late in pregnancy, alternatives should be considered.

Anticonvulsants

The interpretation of studies of anticonvulsants in pregnancy is difficult, since many patients are taking a combination of drugs. A study of 125 women during 133 pregnancies[47] revealed five perinatal deaths, nine infants with structural birth defects, and two with fetal hydantoin syndrome. There was an inverse correlation between maternal serum folate and phenytoin levels. The same workers studied 139 epileptic women through 152 pregnancies[48] and compared them with controls. There was no difference in the incidence of pregnancy induced hypertension or of premature labour, but one infant was stillborn due to placental abruption.

Many congenital abnormalities have been reported in the infants of epileptic mothers. The most common appear to be orofacial cleft deformity and congenital heart disease[49]. The incidence is 2.4 times that in the general population, and abnormalities are more likely if the patient is treated, if the dosage is high, and if more than one drug is used[50,51].

Valproate has been implicated in a 20-fold increased incidence of neural tube defects[52]. Phenytoin has been reported to cause minor congenital defects in up to 30% of infants, and major defects in about 5%[53]. There is also some evidence of a slight decrease in head circumference in the babies of women taking anticonvulsants during pregnancy[54]. This has been confirmed by several other authors[51,55–58].

A large study of 1490 women taking anticonvulsants during pregnancy found four cases of spina bifida, three of which were born to women taking carbamazepine, either alone or in combination with other drugs[59]. In a meta-analysis of 18 studies, the author concludes that the relative risk of spina bifida after carbamazepine *in utero* is almost 14 times the expected rate. Another prospective study documented the outcome of pregnancy in 72 women taking anticonvulsants[60]. The predominant pattern of adverse effects in those on carbamazepine alone included craniofacial defects (11%), fingernail hypoplasia (26%) and developmental delay (20%).

Folic acid supplements to the mother prior to becoming pregnant reduce the risk of neural tube defects in infants at risk[61].

Later in pregnancy, there is a risk of coagulation defect in the infant. The use of vitamin K in the mother prior to delivery, and immediately afterwards in the neonate, has been recommended[62].

A recent risk-benefit assessment of anticonvulsants in women of child-bearing potential[63] concludes that preconceptual counselling is important, that carbamazepine is probably the safest drug to choose, and that women who continue treatment in pregnancy should be offered ultrasound and alpha-fetoprotein evaluation at 16–18 weeks.

Mood Stabilizing Drugs

Valproate and carbamazepine are discussed above.

There have been conflicting reports regarding lithium in pregnancy. A 'lithium baby register' was therefore instituted to collect systematic information regarding babies exposed to lithium *in utero*[64,65]. Eleven per cent of 225 babies were found to have congenital malformations; 3% were relatively minor, but 18 (8%), had malformations involving the heart and great vessels. Somewhat surprisingly, six of the babies had the rare Ebstein's anomaly. The author points out that the study was retrospective, and might have suffered from biased data collection because abnormalities were more likely to be reported than normal children. Other studies have found no such association. No cardiovascular abnormalities were detected in 50 children exposed to lithium *in utero*[66], and another author found that amongst the mothers of 59 children with Ebstein's anomaly, none had taken lithium during pregnancy[67]. Cardiac defects have not been a significant finding in animal teratogenicity studies[68].

There is a theoretical risk of hypothyroidism in the fetus, and the mother's thyroid status should be monitored throughout the pregnancy.

It is also important to remember that the renal clearance of lithium is increased towards the end of pregnancy, and decreases abruptly soon after delivery[69]. Frequent monitoring of lithium levels is required, and the dose may need increasing during the latter part of pregnancy. It is also advisable to lower or discontinue the dose a few days before delivery in order to avoid toxic levels, resuming it a few days later.

Long-term follow up is encouraging. The development of 60 'lithium babies' was compared with that of their siblings who had not been exposed to lithium in fetal life, but had experienced a similar environment[70]. No significant difference was found between the two groups.

Conclusions

Much of the information we have about psychotropic drugs in pregnancy is incomplete or inadequate, relying on individual case reports, or small retrospective studies. These are biased by the fact that abnormalities are more likely to be reported than a normal outcome of pregnancy. The larger epidemiological studies and prospective studies give much more reliable information. In addition, information tends to be disseminated in a wide variety of pharmaceutical, paediatric, obstetric and psychiatric journals, so that it is difficult to access when needed. A few review papers do exist, but rapidly become out of date. However, pharmaceutical manufacturers offer an extremely helpful advisory service by telephone, and will either fax or post relevant papers on request.

Any medication in pregnancy carries a theoretical risk, but this has to be balanced against the very real need for treatment in many cases. Outstanding examples include the schizophrenic patient who is well maintained on depot medication, but who runs a risk of relapse if it is discontinued, the 'brittle' manic-depressive who may relapse whilst trying to become pregnant, and the epileptic mother in whom the risk of maternal fits may be a hazard to both mother and child.

The clinician must be aware of all the information available in order to make an informed decision about the need for medication as opposed to the risk to mother and child if it is withheld. They also need to be able to explain clearly the risks to the mother, and to justify the decision in any medicolegal setting.

Pre-pregnancy counselling is advised for those on antiepileptic medication, and folate supplements can be given before conception. For patients on lithium, it is also helpful to discuss the pros and cons of stopping medication before becoming pregnant. The alternative is to continue medication and to have a specialized scan to visualize the heart chambers at 16 weeks. This implies that the mother will consider termination if there is an abnormality.

It is generally wise to avoid medication wherever possible in the early stages of pregnancy (ie before the 10th week). Drugs about which there is a reliable body of knowledge are to be preferred, the dosage should be kept as low as possible to control symptoms, and the medication given in frequent small doses or, where possible, in depot form in order to avoid high peak levels.

Many patients will present having become pregnant whilst taking psychotropic drugs. If they present early, there is probably some benefit in stopping the medication, but the period of greatest risk is before the 40th day, and the pregnancy may not have been identified by this stage.

All those on psychotropic medication at conception or in the early stages of pregnancy should have alpha-fetoprotein estimations and an early ultrasound scan. Patients on lithium should have frequent serum level estimations and checks on thyroid function.

Later in pregnancy, the clinician's anxiety centres on the effect of the drug on the neonate if maternal serum levels are high. Because the infant's detoxification mechanisms are immature, the effect of the drug on the baby after delivery may be exaggerated or prolonged. Alternatively, as with the phenothiazines and benzodiazepines, withdrawal effects may occur. There is often a need to reduce the maternal dosage in the last few weeks of pregnancy, and the attending paediatrician should always be alerted if a mother is on medication at delivery, in case of adverse effects on the baby.

Psychotropic Drugs in Breast Milk

The psychiatric symptoms and syndromes which may occur in the postpartum period are, as we have seen, many and varied, ranging from the transient weepiness and lability of mood of the 'blues' to the major disturbances of psychotic illness. This in itself creates difficulties for the clinician trying to plan a suitable treatment regimen. When the mother is breast-feeding, this difficulty is compounded by the inadequacy and inaccessibility of information about the transmission of psychotropic drugs in breast milk, and the effect of these drugs on the baby.

In general terms, drugs which pass easily and in high concentrations into breast milk are those which are largely water soluble, do not bind easily to protein molecules, are weakly alkaline, and have a molecular weight of 200 or less. Examples of such drugs include alcohol and tetracyclines. Lipophilic, or fat soluble drugs (which include most psychotropic agents) also pass easily into breast milk by virtue of its high fat content in comparison with plasma.

When the drug has passed from maternal serum into breast milk, other factors must be taken into consideration. The baby's age and weight, the quantity of milk intake, the rate of intestinal absorption and the efficiency of the baby's detoxification mechanisms and renal clearance will all affect the infant's serum level of the drug. Prematurity, neonatal jaundice and congenital enzyme deficiencies will impair the baby's ability to deal with administered drugs. All of the above factors can lead to a build-up of drug concentrations with continuous dosing.

The lack of available information on the subject reflects the reluctance of clinicians to prescribe psychotropic drugs to lactating patients, the reluctance of patients to accept them, and the methodological difficulties of finding sufficient patients to provide meaningful results. Hence much of the existing literature refers to single dose studies. The technical difficulties of assaying drugs at very low concentrations in fluids other than serum, and a general lack of interest from the pharmaceutical industry are also to blame.

Particularly where psychotropic drugs are concerned, whose use at times may be literally life saving, there is a strong case for the systematic investigation of drug concentrations in the breast milk of volunteer patients who do not wish to breast feed. It would be very helpful if this were to be made an obligatory part of the evaluation of all new drugs.

Since the measurements involved are numerous, interpretation and comparison of the reports of different authors can be confusing unless a standard method of reporting is used. The most accurate and informative measurement would seem to be the infant's serum level, as this would take into account the neonate's ability to metabolize and excrete the drug, and include the possibility of accumulation of drugs with a prolonged half-life. However, this assay is invasive and may not be ethically justifiable. An estimation of the milk concentration in standard units, together with a calculation of the daily dose to the infant based on a standard intake of one litre of milk daily, would give useful guidance. This would enable the clinician to calculate the baby's intake in units per kilogram of body weight, and to compare this with the paediatric dosage where this is applicable.

In many cases, the milk/plasma ratio is used as an index, but this is only applicable in 'steady state' conditions, such as continuous intravenous infusion. It may bear little relationship to the levels in intermittent oral dosage, and does not take into account the time lag between maternal and infant absorption, (approximately three hours).

In the interpretation of existing research it is important to note the maternal dose, the time elapsed between dose and sampling, and the duration of action of the drug concerned. In general, single dose studies are less informative than those of prolonged use, as a reasonably steady state plasma level should be achieved in the mother, and the possibility of accumulation of the drug taken into account. Some researchers estimate the drug levels only; but those which also estimate the levels of active metabolites are clearly more helpful.

Where infant serum levels are quoted, the age and weight of the baby are important factors to note. Although clinical assessment of the infant at the time may be reassuring, it is not possible to rule out subtle or remote effects on the infant without long-term follow-up.

The following are possible manoeuvres to prevent adverse

effects on the breast-fed infant:

- delay therapy until weaning has taken place

- avoid drugs about which there is no information about breast milk transmission

- choose drugs which have low concentrations in milk

- avoid breast-feeding at times of peak drug concentration in the mother

- administer the drug to the mother before the baby's longest sleep period

- if the administration of the drug is likely to be over a short period, breast-feeding can be discontinued pro tem. but the milk supply preserved by the use of a breast pump.

Major Tranquillizers

Chlorpromazine

The results of single dose studies, such as that of Blacker *et al.*[71], suggest that, even after a maternal dose of 1200 mg, the amount received by the baby would be negligible. Two hours after medication the milk concentration was shown to be 290 ng/ml, which is well below the paediatric dose. The authors state that there was no detectable drug in the milk after a dose of 600 mg twice daily to the mother. However, other authors[72] report that the milk concentration in a woman taking 200 mg chlorpromazine daily for seven days was 40–150 ng/ml, giving the infant a daily dose of 4–15 mg. The infant suffered no ill effects.

This discrepancy in levels is perhaps explained by the work of Wiles *et al*[73], who showed that maternal serum and milk levels vary widely while on a constant dose. The levels of chlorpromazine and its metabolites in the plasma of four nursing mothers varied from 16 to 52 ng/ml, and in the milk from 7 to 98 ng/ml. Two of these mothers breast-fed; one infant who absorbed milk containing 92 ng/ml was reported as being drowsy. Unfortunately, no information is given regarding the maternal dose or the time lapse between administration and sampling.

Three early studies[17,18,74] examined the long-term effect on children of maternal chlorpromazine given during lactation. Although no details of dosage are given, some of these children were followed up for as long as five years, and no adverse physical or developmental effects were noted. Nevertheless, animal studies have shown that early postnatal administration of chlorpromazine can produce behavioural changes in the young[75].

Haloperidol

A single case report[76] states that a mother taking 30 mg of haloperidol daily produced breast milk with a concentration of 5 ng/ml and that this level fell to 2 ng/ml when the maternal dose was reduced to 12 mg/day. They calculated that the baby's maximum intake would be in the order of 0.0075 mg daily. However, Whalley et al.[77] showed that larger amounts, up to 23 ng/ml, were excreted in the milk of a mother taking 10 mg haloperidol daily. In spite of this, the three-week-old infant was not sedated, fed well, and continued to thrive. She was also reported to have achieved all her developmental milestones at six and 12 months of age.

The serum levels of haloperidol are known to vary widely in adult patients, and it would be unwise to assume safety on the basis of two single case study reports.

Other oral neuroleptics

Thioridazine (Melleril) is an unsuitable drug for nursing mothers on account of the occasional incidence of blood dyscrasias.

Trifluoperazine (Stelazine) has been examined only in animal studies[78,79].

Flupenthixol (Depixol, Fluanxol) has been investigated in one patient taking 2 mg/day. The milk concentrations were found to be approximately 30% higher than those in maternal serum[4]. On a daily consumption of one litre of milk, the baby's intake would be in the order of 0.002 mg, which is equivalent to an adult dose of 0.04 mg/day. Other authors[80] have found that the infant might ingest approximately 1–2% of the maternal dose.

Two studies of zuclopenthixol (Clopixol)[80,81] have found milk/plasma ratios varying from 0.12 to 0.85.

Sulpiride (Dolmatil, Sulpitil) and its isomers were given at a dose of 100 mg daily for five days postpartum to nursing mothers to improve lactation[82]. The mean fifth day concentration of sulpiride in milk was 830 ng/ml, and no serious side-effects were noted in the mothers or children. No long-term observations were made on these children.

Depot medication

In the case of the long-acting phenothiazines, fluphenazine enanthate (Moditen) and fluphenazine decanoate (Modecate), the maternal serum levels are in general very low, and it is only recently that sufficiently sensitive methods have been available for serum assay.

There is one case report[5] of a patient who received 50 mg fluphenazine decanoate every three weeks during and after her pregnancy. The baby was breast-fed for only five days, but, at four weeks of age, developed minor extrapyramidal symptoms. The baby was said to be healthy two months after delivery, and the mother's account of the child at 20 months of age was equally reassuring.

Four patients given intramuscular flupenthixol decanoate (Depixol) in doses ranging from 30 to 60 mg every two weeks, have been studied[4]. As with the oral medication, the breast milk concentrations were higher than in maternal serum, but the total daily intake for the baby was low.

No information is available for pipothiazine palmitate (Piportil), or pimozide (Orap), but the manufacturers suggest that neither should be used in lactating mothers.

Conclusions

Neuroleptic medication is used in the treatment of florid psychotic states in the puerperium. In such cases, breast-feeding is often impractical anyway, but, if it is to be continued, the medication should be kept at as low a level as is compatible with control of the mother's mental state. The medication of choice is that which has available information concerning breast milk levels; the manufacturer should be asked if it is possible to estimate maternal serum and breast milk concentrations in the individual patient.

Patients receiving depot medication are usually those suffering from chronic psychoses in whom the drug has been administered throughout pregnancy. In such cases, the fetus has already been exposed to the medication *in utero*, and it is likely that a few more weeks of exposure is no more harmful than sudden withdrawal at the time of delivery. However, it is possible that there is a differential excretion of neuroleptic and anti-Parkinsonian medication in breast milk, and the infant must be monitored carefully for signs of extrapyramidal dysfunction.

Antidepressants

Tricyclics

There is a good deal of conflicting evidence as far as this group of drugs is concerned. Several authors[83-85] have stated that imipramine (Tofranil) could not be detected in breast milk even after five days of oral treatment to the mother. Another[86] found that only a small fraction of the maternal plasma concentration is found in breast milk. In contrast, a more recent study[87] has found that the concentrations of imipramine and its active metabolite, desipramine, were similar in breast milk and maternal plasma. Although the latter study referred only to a single case, the estimations were made after a daily dose of 200 mg for 16 days, and therefore resembled more closely the situation in clinical practice. In spite of this high dose, it was reported that the maternal serum level was well below the therapeutic range, and that the mother showed no clinical response.

Other authors[88] have calculated that, if the maternal serum levels of imipramine and desipramine together are 200 ng/ml (a therapeutic level) and the breast milk concentration is similar, then a 5 kg infant taking one litre of milk daily will receive a total daily dose of about 0.2 mg of the combined tricyclics (ie about 0.04 mg/kg). They compare this favourably with the recommended dose for older children of 1.0 mg/kg, but the comparison is not justifiable because of the immaturity of the detoxification mechanisms in neonates.

Maternal doses of amitriptyline (Domical, Lentizol, Tryptizol) of up to 150 mg/day for three weeks produced a maternal serum level of 238 ng/ml and no detectable amount (ie less than 28 ng/ml) in the infant's serum[88]. Simultaneous blood and milk samples were obtained in one study from a woman who had been taking 75 mg sustained release amitriptyline daily for two weeks[89]. No active drug could be detected in the infant's serum and the four-month-old child was said to be unaffected. Similarly, a patient on 100 mg of amitriptyline daily had comparable levels in maternal serum and milk at six weeks postpartum, but none could be detected in the infant's serum[90].

Nortriptyline (Allegron, Aventyl) has been examined in the serum of seven depressed mothers and their babies after a minimum of 15 days at a steady oral dose[91]. The maternal concentrations ranged from 47 to 164 ng/ml, and none was detected in the infants' serum. There was no evidence of accumulation of the drug in the infants on prolonged breast-feeding, and no adverse effects were reported in the babies.

Desipramine (Pertofran) and its metabolites were measured in milk and maternal and infant plasma during administration of 300 mg/day to the mother[92]. None could be detected in the infant's plasma, and no signs of toxicity in the baby were seen after three weeks of treatment.

Dothiepin (Prothiaden) levels were assayed in the milk of two lactating mothers[93]. In one, on a dose of 75 mg daily for three months, the serum level was 33 ng/ml and the milk level 11 ng/ml. A second patient, who had received 300 mg dothiepin intermittently over a six-day period, showed levels of 10 ng/ml in serum and milk. It was calculated that the infant would receive only 1/650 of an adult dose, but no metabolites were measured. A more recent study has measured dothiepin and its metabolites in eight women on varying doses of the drug[94]. The authors calculate that the infants received 0.58% of the daily maternal dose for dothiepin, but up to 2.47% of one of its metabolites. However the infants' serum levels were generally so low as to be unmeasurable, and no adverse effects were reported in the babies.

A recent clinical study looking at 20 breast-feeding mothers with postnatal depression and treated with tricyclic drugs, found no developmental delay in any of the babies who were followed up for a maximum of three years. This study reveals the hazards of not giving medication; all five of the mothers refusing medication continued to be depressed, two were admitted to hospital and required ECT, and the remainder were so severely ill that they later stopped breast-feeding in order to take medication[95].

Heterocyclics

The manufacturers of Bolvidon (mianserin) state that, in animal studies, only 0.1% of the adult dose is transmitted to the nursling (Organon Laboratories, personal communication, 1993). In a recent study of two lactating women, approximately 1.4% of the adult oral dose was found in milk after a maternal dose of 60 mg for nine days, and 0.5% after 40 mg for 14 days[96]. The occasional occurrence of blood dyscrasias in adults suggests that it would be wise to avoid this medication in nursing mothers.

Another tetracyclic drug, maprotiline hydrochloride (Ludiomil) highlights the hazards of extrapolating the results of tests on one drug to others in the same group. This compound is strongly lipophilic, and the concentration in breast milk is 30–50% higher than in maternal plasma. It is not recommended for nursing mothers[97,98].

Amoxapine (Asendis) has been shown to pass into breast milk in a single patient. The infant dose was calculated as less than 0.07% of the maternal dose[99].

Monoamine oxidase inhibitors
Two authors[84,85] assert that therapeutic doses of tranylcypromine (Parnate) are secreted in breast milk in doses too small to affect the child. Another[100] states that no ill effects have been noted in the infants of mothers taking isocarboxazid (Marplan), but goes on to say that animal studies on nialamide (Niamid) have shown that the maturation of young is affected, and that there is a high mortality rate in the offspring. In view of the potential for interaction of this group of drugs with other medication or dietary factors, it would be unwise to continue breast-feeding while taking this group of drugs.

The most recent member of this group, moclobemide (Manerix) is a reversible monoamine oxidase-A inhibitor (MAOI) without the need for the strict dietary restrictions of the old MAOIs. A single report on six women given a single dose showed that approximately 1% of the adult dose would be transmitted to the baby[101].

Selective serotonin uptake inhibitors
The 5-HT reuptake inhibitors are very suitable for the postnatally depressed mother on account of the lack of sedative side-effects and relatively rapid antidepressant response. Unfortunately, little is known about the infant effects through breast-feeding.

The manufacturers of paroxetine (Seroxat) state that the drug is found in the milk of nursing mothers at a concentration similar to that in maternal serum. They infer that less than 1% of the daily maternal dose would be transmitted to the infant (Smith, Kline Beecham, 1993, personal communication). There are two anecdotal reports of abnormal behaviour in a breast-fed infant whose mother was taking paroxetine. One baby was described as being 'jittery', and the second was irritable at night.

Fluoxetine (Prozac) and its metabolites were measured in the serum and milk of a patient on 20 mg daily for 53 days[102]. The dose to the infant was estimated at 15–20 µg/kg daily. The medication was commenced at five weeks' postpartum and the baby was developing normally at four months.

Plasma levels of fluoxetine and its metabolites were investigated in another mother after two months on 20 mg daily[103]. Plasma levels were 100.5 ng/ml fluoxetine and 194.5 ng/ml norfluoxetine. The corresponding milk levels were 28.8 ng/ml and 41.6 ng/ml. The baby was thought to be somewhat irritable for two weeks after the drug was started, but was thriving at five months.

Other antidepressants
Information on viloxazine (Vivalan) is limited to a single study of one patient who took 300 mg daily for two days (JR Holmes, 1977, internal publication, Fairmile Hospital). The concentration in breast milk was 10–20% of that in maternal serum. This drug, which is chemically distinct from the tri- and tetracyclics, is probably unsuitable for nursing mothers.

Trazodone hydrochloride (Molipaxin) which is also chemically distinct from the tricyclics and tetracyclics, produced low drug concentrations in milk after a single dose[104], but the effects of the drug on the infant have not been studied.

Conclusions
No current agreement exists about the advisability of therapy with antidepressants during lactation. Even though immediate side-effects in the infant appear to be minimal, long-term effects on the child's neurological and behavioural development cannot be reliably ruled out. However, this anxiety has to be weighed against the child's development in the care of a depressed mother.

Certainly the MOAIs and the 5-HT reuptake inhibitors should currently be avoided, although it is hoped that there will be further information on the latter in the near future. Tricyclics carry the greatest volume of clinical experience and experimental data, and are undoubtedly the safest at present. Infant effects can be minimized by giving a secondary amine (desipramine or nortriptyline), and by giving the whole dose at bedtime and bottle-feeding during the night. The baby should be carefully monitored for immediate and long-term adverse effects.

Hypnotics and Sedatives

Barbiturates
These are rarely used at the present time, but the exception that is important in psychiatric practice is the use of intravenous anaesthesia prior to ECT. This appears to cause low levels in breast milk, and there are no adverse effects reported in the infant[105].

Benzodiazepines
This group of drugs should generally be avoided in the puerperium because of the potential for addiction, escalation of the dose, and, in particular, where the care of infants is concerned, disinhibition in a depressed or anxious mother. Breast milk has been shown to contain small amounts of benzodiazepine-like substances[106]. Thus we can infer that the infant has benzodiazepine receptors, but it does not mean that administration of the drug to the mother is safe. Indeed, the longer-acting members of this group of drugs can accumulate in the baby, particularly where the neonate is premature, and has immature detoxification mechanisms, or is jaundiced.

Adverse effects have been shown in infants, both during prolonged administration to the mother, and on abrupt withdrawal[107-109]. Breast-feeding should be avoided for six to eight hours after a single large dose of diazepam (Valium), for example, in the treatment of epilepsy or prior to endoscopy. The use of these drugs is rarely essential, but, if considered to be so, the shorter-acting drugs such as oxazepam or lorazepam are to be preferred[110-113]. A comparison of nitrazepam (Mogadon, Somnite) with a half-life of 24 hours, with midazolam (Hypnovel) which has a two-hour half-life, showed that nitrazepam levels in milk increased over the five-day period of administration to the mother because of accumulation of the drug[114]. In contrast, no measurable concentrations of midazolam could be detected in milk.

Temazepam (Normison) is commonly given as a night sedative in postnatal wards. This drug and its metabolite, oxazepam, were measured in the plasma and milk of ten women given 10–20 mg at night within the first 15 days postpartum[115]. The mean milk plasma ratio was less than 0.18, lower than that for diazepam, lorazepam (Ativan) and clonazepam (Rivotril).

Other hypnotics
Chloral hydrate (Noctec, Welldorm) and its metabolites are transferred into breast milk at relatively high levels and may cause sedation in the infant. Both also have a long half-life, and may have a cumulative effect[116,117].

Anticonvulsants

Carbamazepine
Both the original drug and its metabolites are excreted in breast milk, and can be measured in the infant's plasma. Levels are generally low, and no dose-related adverse effects have been reported[118-121]. One case of cholestatic hepatitis, which was reversible on stopping the drug, has been reported[122]. This was probably an idiosyncratic reaction. Close observation of the baby and occasional infant plasma level estimations are recommended.

Clonazepam
One case of infant apnoea has been recorded in relation to maternal use of this drug, but, in general, the infant plasma levels are low[123,124]. Monitoring of the baby's plasma levels may be necessary if there are signs of hypotonia or poor feeding.

Ethosuxamide
The infant's plasma levels of the drug may approximate the therapeutic range, and should be monitored regularly. Some infants have been noted to be drowsy[118,125-127]. Maternal levels should be kept as low as possible within the therapeutic range.

Phenytoin
This is excreted into milk in small amounts, since it has a high affinity for protein, and is weakly acid[128,129]. It is generally tolerated well by breast-fed babies, but occasional idiosyncratic reactions, such as methaemoglobinaemia and cyanosis, have been reported[130].

Primidone
Many of the metabolites of this drug also appear in breast milk, together with large amounts of the drug itself[118,131]. Feeding difficulties have been reported[132], but abrupt withdrawal at birth also appears to have adverse effects[118,129]. Infant plasma levels and infant behaviour should be closely monitored. Abrupt weaning should also be avoided[133].

Valproate
Valproate levels are generally low in breast milk. No adverse effects have been noted in breast-fed infants[134,135].

Conclusions
These drugs occasionally produce mild drowsiness in the infant, but, if the mother was on the medication during pregnancy, breast-feeding can reduce abrupt withdrawal effects in the infant at birth. Infant plasma monitoring is important in babies who show drowsiness, who feed poorly, or who fail to gain weight.

Valproate or carbamazepine are probably the safest of the anticonvulsant group, but plasma monitoring of the baby may be indicated. The dose to the baby can be minimized by giving the total dose at bedtime and bottle-feeding during the night.

Mood Stabilizing Drugs

Lithium
Lithium salts given to the mother pass into milk, at a concentration of 30–50% of that in maternal plasma[136]. In the case of women taking lithium throughout pregnancy, the infant's serum level is approximately 50% of the mother's in the first week of life, falling to 30% in subsequent weeks.

It has been reasoned that the infant has already been exposed to high plasma levels *in utero*, and the absorption from breast milk will produce lower and safer levels[66]. This view is supported by a study of a woman taking 400 mg of lithium carbonate daily at parturition[137]. At delivery, the infant's serum level was similar to her own, but fell postpartum in spite of a doubling of the dose to the mother and the establishment of breast-feeding. Although the lithium concentration in milk almost doubled from the 14th to the 28th day postpartum, the baby's serum level remained relatively constant during the same period. A recent investigation by the author showed that the serum level of a mother on 800 mg lithium citrate daily for 14 days was 0.7 meq/l, whilst that of the totally breast-fed and thriving five-month old baby was 0.03 meq/l.

However, there are two reports of high serum levels in infants whose mothers were on a constant dose of lithium during pregnancy and labour[138,139]. Both infants were cyanosed and hypotonic, but later follow-up on one child was reassuring. Another case demonstrates the possible hazards if the child is ill. A lithium treated mother breast-fed her baby satisfactorily for two months until the child became ill with a cold. Signs of toxicity developed in the infant, whose serum lithium was 1.4 mmol/l, twice that of the mother[140].

There is also a theoretical risk that the infant's bone formation and thyroid function may be compromised by lithium given early in the neonatal period.

Clearly it is unwise to breast-feed a baby who is premature or of low birth weight. Even in a healthy full-term baby it is important to monitor the infant's serum level from time to time, and immediately if there are any signs of toxicity. It will also be necessary to discontinue breast-feeding if the baby becomes ill or dehydrated. In view of the rapid changes of blood volume around parturition, it may also be wise to lower the maternal dose immediately before and after delivery.

Carbamazepine and valproate
These drugs have already been considered in the section on anticonvulsants.

Calcium-channel blockers
These drugs are only occasionally used as mood stabilizers, but, in view of the anxieties about lithium and carbamazepine in the puerperium, they warrant further exploration in the treatment of manic-depressive puerperal psychosis. Several case reports

suggest that verapamil and norverapamil levels are low in milk and infant plasma[141-144].

Beta-adrenergic Blocking Drugs

Both propranolol and labetalol are excreted in small amounts in breast milk. Certainly, in the low doses used in panic disorder, both are probably safe in lactation, even in the early neonatal period. One study showed that a single dose of 40 mg of propranolol to the mother resulted in peak plasma levels of 18–23 ng/ml and milk levels of 4–9 ng/ml[145]. There is a single case report of adverse effects in the infant of a mother taking atenolol[146], and it is important to monitor the infant for signs of bradycardia and respiratory distress.

Hormones

Contraceptives
Breast-feeding in itself inhibits ovulation, but, where it is essential for the mother's mental health for her not to become pregnant again within a short space of time, contraception may be indicated.

Combined oral contraceptives, particularly those with a high oestrogen content, may reduce lactation[147,148], whereas the progesterone-only pill may enhance milk production[149]. Neither oestrogen nor progesterone are secreted in large amounts in breast milk[150-152], but there are isolated reports of breast enlargement in the nursing infants of mothers on the combined oral contraceptive[153,154]. Long-term follow-up has revealed no adverse effects on children up to eight years of age[155].

Progesterone
High doses of progesterone in the early puerperium have been suggested as a suitable prophylactic against the recurrence of postpartum depression[156], and for the treatment of the premenstrual syndrome[157]. In neither case has its efficacy been confirmed in double-blind trials, and the effect on the nursing infant has not been investigated.

Thyroid hormone
Transient hypothyroidism is relatively common in the postnatal period, and often does not require treatment. However, when it

is severe, and thought to be contributing to the mother's mental state, treatment may be indicated. Hypothyroidism may also occur as an adverse effect of lithium therapy. Where mood stabilizing treatment is thought to be essential, and no suitable alternative is thought to be practicable, lithium may be continued with the addition of thyroid replacement therapy. Occasionally thyroxine is also used as an adjunct to antidepressant therapy in resistant cases.

Replacement L-thyroxine treatment providing adequate physiological levels in the mother is unlikely to lead to excessive doses to the baby. L-thyroxine is poorly excreted in breast milk, but liothyronine (Tertroxin) passes into milk more easily and should be avoided[158–161].

Antithyroid agents

In the rare cases of postpartum thyrotoxicosis which warrant treatment, propylthiouracil has low concentrations in breast milk, and does not affect nursing infants[162]. Methimazole and carbimazole pass into breast milk more easily and should be avoided[162–164]. However, the infant's thyroid function should be measured at regular intervals.

Summary

It is clear that much more information is urgently needed regarding the breast milk concentrations of both psychotropics and other drugs that women may need in the puerperium. It seems that most psychotropic drugs are secreted in breast milk, but the crucial question is whether they are present in sufficient quantities to affect the breast-fed infant, either at the time of administration or later in the child's development.

The difficulties lie not only in measuring the drugs in breast milk, but also in interpreting the results. It must be remembered that the neonate is a rapidly changing entity, and the manner in which drugs can be tolerated, detoxified and excreted can vary, not only between individuals, but also in the same individual over a period of time.

No drug administered to the lactating mother can be entirely without risk to her baby, especially if the infant's health is jeopardized in some other way, for example, by prematurity, congenital enzyme deficiency, intercurrent illness, or jaundice, which can impair liver detoxification mechanisms.

However, the advantages of breast-feeding are self-evident, and include the transmission of passive immunity, the avoidance of obesity and food allergies in the infant, and, above all, the facilitation of bonding between mother and child. The importance of breast-feeding to a psychiatrically disturbed mother may be even greater, reinforcing her feelings of capability as a mother, counteracting some of the guilt associated with depressive illness, and helping her to overcome a sense of detachment from reality.

In the drug treatment of puerperal psychiatric illness, no universal rule can apply. Each case requires delicate judgement on the part of the clinician, weighing the benefits of treatment and continued breast-feeding against the inherent risks of untreated mental illness or the disadvantages of ending lactation.

For the minor psychiatric illnesses of the puerperium which are likely to resolve spontaneously, or to respond to other forms of treatment such as counselling, psychotherapy or practical interventions, only the most trivial risk to the baby can be acceptable. In the case of the florid forms of puerperal illness, in which harm to the mother or child may result from failure to treat, or in chronic psychotic illness, very likely to relapse if treatment is withdrawn, the need for medication is paramount.

When medication is used in lactating mothers, it is advisable to ask the manufacturer to analyse plasma and milk samples for both the drug itself and its metabolites, and to publish these details in the data sheet. This would be of invaluable help to those having to make decisions in the future.

Most importantly, it is mandatory to monitor the health and development of all infants exposed to maternal drugs, not only at the time of exposure, but also over a prolonged period.

References

1. Hill RM, Desmond MM and Kay JI. (1966) Extrapyramidal dysfunction in an infant of a schizophrenic mother. *Journal of Pediatrics*. **69**: 589–95.

2. Tamer A, McKey R, Arias D, *et al*. (1969) Phenothiazine induced extrapyramidal dysfunction in the neonate. *Journal of Pediatrics*. **75**: 479–90.

3. Levy W and Wisniewsky K. (1974) Chlorpromazine causing extrapyramidal dysfunction. *New York State Journal of Medicine*. **74**: 684–5.

4. Kirk L and Jorgensen A. (1980) Concentrations of cis(Z)-flupenthixol in maternal serum, amniotic fluid, umbilical cord serum and milk. *Psychopharmacology*. **72**: 107–8.

5. Cleary MF. (1977) Fluphenazine decanaote during pregnancy. *American Journal of Psychiatry*. **134**: 815–6.

6. Rumeau-Rouquette C, Goujard J and Huel G. (1977) Possible teratogenic effect of phenothiazines in human beings. *Teratology*. **15**: 57–64.

7. Slone D, Suskind V, Heinonen OP, *et al*. (1977) Antenatal exposure to the phenothiazines in relation to congenital malformations, perinatal mortality, birth weight and IQ score. *American Journal of Obstetrics and Gynecology*. **128**: 486–8.

8. Edlund MJ and Craig TJ. (1984) Antipsychotic drug use and birth defects: An epidemiologic reassessment. *Comprehensive Psychiatry*. **25**: 32–7.

9. Rieder RO, Rosenthal D, Wender P, *et al*. (1975) The offspring of schizophrenics – foetal and neonatal deaths. *Archives of General Psychiatry*. **32**: 200–11.

10. Sobel DE. (1960) Foetal damage due to ECT, insulin coma, chlorpromazine or reserpine. *Archives of General Psychiatry*. **2**: 606–11.

11. Van Waes A and Van der Velde EJ. (1969) Safety evaluation of haloperidol in the treatment of hyperemesis gravidarum. *Journal of Clinical Pharmacology*. **9**: 224–7.

12. Rawlings WJ, Ferguson R and Madison TG. (1963) Phenmetrazine and trifluoperazine. *Medical Journal of Australia*. **1**: 370.

13. Moriarty AK and Nance MR. (1963) Trifluoperazine and pregnancy. *Canadian Medical Association Journal*. **88**: 375–6.

14. Goldberg HL and DiMascio A. (1978) Psychotropic drugs in pregnancy. In: (Lipton MA, DiMascio A and Killan KF, editors.) *Psychopharmacology: A generation of progress*. Raven Press, New York.

15. Ananth J. (1975) Congenital malformations with psychopharmacologic agents. *Comprehensive Psychiatry*. **16**: 437–45.

16. Kris EB. (1965) Children of mothers maintained on pharmacotherapy during pregnancy and postpartum. *Current Therapeutic Research*. **7**: 785–9.

17. Kris LB and Carmichael DM. (1957) Chlorpromazine maintenance therapy during pregnancy and confinement. *Psychiatric Quarterly*. **31**: 690–5.

18. Kris EB. (1962) Children born to mothers on pharmacotherapy during pregnancy and postpartum. *Recent Advances in Biological Psychiatry*. **4**: 180–7.

19. Nishimura H and Tanimura T. (1976) *Clinical aspects of the teratogenicity of drugs*. Elsevier, New York.

20. Barson AJ. (1972) Malformed infants. *British Medical Journal*. **ii**: 45.

21. Morrow AW. (1972) Limb deformities associated with iminodibenzyl hydrochloride. *Medical Journal of Australia*. **1**: 658–9.

22. Crombie DL, Pinsent RJ, Fleming D, *et al.* (1975) Fetal effects of tranquillisers in pregnancy. *New England Journal of Medicine*. **293**: 198–9.

23. Kuenssberg EV and Knox JD. (1972) Imipramine in pregnancy. *British Medical Journal*. **ii**: 292.

24. Idanpaan-Heikkila J and Saxen L. (1973) Possible teratogenicity of imipramine-chloropyramine. *Lancet*. **ii**: 282–4.

25. Webster PAC. (1973) Withdrawal symptoms in neonates associated with maternal antidepressant therapy. *Lancet.* **ii**: 318–19.

26. Shearer WT, Shreiner RL and Marshall RE. (1972) Urinary retention in a neonate secondary to maternal ingestion of nortriptyline. *Journal of Pediatrics.* **81**: 570–2.

27. Zahle Ostergaard G and Pedersen SE. (1982) Neonatal effects of maternal clomipramine treatment. *Pediatrics.* **69**: 233–4.

28. Poulson E and Robson JM. (1964) Effect of phenelzine and some related compounds on pregnancy. *Journal of Endocrinology.* **30**: 205–15.

29. Dorner G, Heicht K and Hinz G. (1976) Teratopsychogenic effects apparently produced by nonphysiological neurotransmitter concentrations during brain differentiation. *Endokrinologie.* **68**: 323–30.

30. Dorner G, Staudt J, Wenzel J, *et al.* (1977) Further evidence of teratogenic effects apparently produced by brain transmitters during brain differentiation. *Endokrinologie.* **70**: 326–30.

31. Baldwin JA, Davidson EJ, Pritchard AL, *et al.* (1989) The reproductive toxicology of paroxetine. *Acta Psychiatrica Scandinavica.* **80**(suppl. 350): 37–9.

32. Pastuszak A, Schick-Boschetto B, Zuber C, *et al.* (1993) Pregnancy outcome following first trimester exposure to fluoxetine. *JAMA.* **269**: 2246–8.

33. Edwards JG, Inman WHW, Wilson L, *et al.* (1994) Prescription-event monitoring of 10 401 patients treated with fluvoxamine. *British Journal of Psychiatry.* **164**: 387–95.

34. Safra MJ and Oakley GP. (1975) Association between cleft lip with or without cleft palate and prenatal exposure to diazepam. *Lancet*: **ii**: 478–80.

35. Saxen I and Saxen L. (1975) Association between maternal intake of diazepam and oral clefts. *Lancet.* **ii**: 498.

36. Aarskog D. (1975) Association between maternal intake of diazepam and oral clefts. *Lancet.* **ii**: 921.

37. Bergman U, Rosa FW, Baum C, *et al.* (1992) Effects of exposure to benzodiazepines during fetal life. *Lancet.* **340**: 694–6.

38. Milkovitch L and Van den Berg BJ. (1974) Effects of prenatal meprobamate and chlordiazepoxide hydrochloride on human embryonic and foetal development. *New England Journal of Medicine.* **291**: 1268–71.

39. Hartz SC, Heinonen OP, Shapiro S, *et al.* (1975) Antenatal exposure to meprobamate and chordiazepoxide in relation to malformations, mental development and childhood mortality. *New England Journal of Medicine.* **292**: 726–8.

40. Greenberg G, Inman WHW, Weatherall JAC, *et al.* (1977) Maternal drug histories and congenital abnormalities. *British Medical Journal.* **ii**: 853–6.

41. Laegreid L, Conradi N, Hagberg G, *et al.* (1992) Psychotropic drug use in pregnancy and perinatal death. *Acta Obstetrica et Gynecolica Scandinavica.* **71**: 451–7.

42. Cree JE, Meyer J and Hailey DM. (1973) Diazepam in labour: Its metabolism and effect on the clinical condition and thermogenesis of the newborn. *British Medical Journal.* **iv**: 251–5.

43. Haram K and Bakke OM. (1980) Diazepam as an induction agent for caesarian section: A clinical and pharmacokinetic study of foetal drug exposure. *British Journal of Obstetrics and Gynaecology.* **87**: 506–12.

44. Beeley L. (1981) Adverse effects of drugs in later pregnancy. *Clinics in Obstetrics and Gynecology.* **8**: 275–90.

45. Rementeria JL and Bhatt K. (1977) Withdrawal symptoms in neonates from intrauterine exposure to diazepam. *Journal of Pediatrics.* **90**: 123–6.

46. Pakshi A, Pierog SH, Nigam SK, *et al.* (1976) Chlordiazepoxide withdrawal in the neonate. *American Journal of Obstetrics and Gynecology.* **124**: 212–13.

47. Hiilesmaa VK, Teramo R and Granstrom M-L. (1983) Serum folate concentrations in women with epilepsy. *British Medical Journal.* **287**: 577–9.

48. Hiilesmaa VK, Bardy A and Teramo R. (1985) Obstetric outcome in women with epilepsy. *American Journal of Obstetrics and Gynecology.* **152**: 499–504.

49. Fedrick J. (1983) Epilepsy and pregnancy: A report from the Oxford Record Linkage Study. *British Medical Journal.* **ii**: 442–8.

50. Dansky L, Anderman E, Sherwin AI, *et al.* (1980) Maternal epilepsy and congenital malformations: Correlation with maternal plasma anticonvulsant levels. *Epilepsy, Pregnancy and the Child* (Janz D, *et al.* editors.) Raven Press, New York, 251–8.

51. Lindhout D, Hoppener RJ and Meinardi H. (1984) Teratogenicity of antiepileptic drug combinations. *Epilepsia.* **25**: 77–83.

52. Lindhout D and Schmidt D. (1986) *In-utero* exposure to valproate and neural tube defects. *Lancet.* **i**: 1392–3.

53. Beuhler BA. (1985) Epoxide hydrolase activity and foetal hydantoin syndrome. *Clinical Research.* **33**: A129.

54. Hiilesmaa VK, Teramo K, Granstrom ML, *et al.* (1981) Head growth retardation associated with maternal antiepileptic drugs. *Lancet.* **ii**: 165–7.

55. Kaneko S, Fukushima Y, Sato T, *et al.* (1982) Fetal head growth retardation due to maternal antiepileptic drug use. *Brain and Nerve.* **34**: 705–11.

56. Otani K, Fukushima Y, *et al.* (1988) Teratogenicity of antiepileptic drugs: Analysis of possible risk factors. *Epilepsia.* **29**: 459–67.

57. Deblay MF, Vert P and Andre M. (1982) Infants of epileptic mothers. *Nouvelle Presse Médicale.* **11**: 173–6.

58. Koch S, Goepfert-Geyer I, Jaegar-Roman E, *et al.* (1983) Anticonvulsants during pregnancy: A prospective study on the course of pregnancy, malformation and child development. *Deutsche Medizinische Wochenschrift.* **108**: 250–7.

59. Rosa FW. (1991) Spina bifida in women treated with carbamazepine during pregnancy. *New England Journal of Medicine.* **324**: 674–7.

60. Jones KL, Lacro RV, Johnson KA, *et al.* (1989) Pattern of malformations in the children of women treated with carbamazepine during pregnancy. *New England Journal of Medicine.* **320**: 1661–6.

61. MRC Vitamin Study Research Group. (1991) Prevention of neural tube defects: Results of the Medical Research Council vitamin study. *Lancet.* **338**: 131–7.

62. Manderbrot L, Guillaumont M, LeClerq M, *et al.* (1988) Placental transfer of vitamin K and its implications in foetal haemostasis. *Thrombosis and Haemostasis.* **60**: 39–43.

63. O'Brien MD and Gilmour-White S. (1993) Epilepsy and pregnancy. *British Medical Journal.* **307**: 492–5.

64. Schou M, Goldfield MD, Weinstein MR, *et al.* (1973) Lithium and pregnancy. I: Report from the register of lithium babies. *British Medical Journal.* **ii**: 135–6.

65. Schou M and Weinstein MR. (1980) Problems of maintenance treatment during pregnancy delivery and lactation. *Aggressologie.* **21A**: 7–9.

66. Cunniff CM, Sahn DJ, Reed KL, *et al.* (1989) Pregnancy outcome in women treated with lithium. *Teratology.* **39**: 447–8.

67. Zalzstein E, Koren G, Einarson T, *et al.* (1990) A case-control study of the association between first trimester exposure to lithium and Ebstein's anomaly. *American Journal of Cardiology.* **65**: 817–18.

68. Schou M. (1990) Lithium treatment during pregnancy, delivery and lactation: An update. *Journal of Clinical Psychiatry.* **51**: 410–13.

69. Schou M, Amdisen A and Steenstrup OR. (1973) Lithium in pregnancy. II: Hazards to women given lithium during pregnancy and lactation. *British Medical Journal.* **ii**: 137–8.

70. Schou M. (1976) What happened later to the lithium babies? *Acta Psychiatrica Scandinavica.* **54**: 193–7.

71. Blacker KH, Weinstein BD and Ellman G. (1962) Mothers' milk and chlorpromazine. *American Journal of Psychiatry.* **119**: 178–9.

72. Uhlif F and Ryznar J. (1973) The appearance of chlorpromazine in mothers' milk. *Activitas Nervosa Superior (Praha).* **15**: 106.

73. Wiles DH, Orr MW and Kolakowska T. (1978) Chlorpromazine levels in plasma and milk of nursing mothers. *British Journal of Clinical Pharmacology.* **5**: 272–3.

74. Ayd F. (1964) Children born of mothers treated with chlorproma-
     zine during pregnancy. *Clinical Medicine*. **71**: 1758–63.

75. Leonard BE. (1983) Behavioural teratology and toxicology. In:
     (Grahame-Smith DG and Cowen P, editors.) *Psychopharmacol-
     ogy*. Excerpta Medica, Amsterdam, 248–99.

76. Stewart RB, Karas B and Springer PK. (1980) Haloperidol excre-
     tion in human milk. *American Journal of Psychiatry*. **137**: 849–50.

77. Whalley LJ, Blain PG and Prime JK. (1981) Haloperidol secreted
     in breast milk. *British Medical Journal*. **ii**: 1746–7.

78. Flanagan TL, Lin TH, Novick WJ, *et al*. (1959) Spectrophoto-
     metric method for the determination of chlorpromazine and
     chlorpromazine sulphoxide in biological fluids. *Journal of Medi-
     cinal and Pharmaceutical Chemistry*. **1**: 263–73.

79. Wilson JT, Brown RD, Cherek DR, *et al*. (1980) Drug excretion in
     human breast milk. *Clinical Pharmacokinetics*. **5**: 1–66.

80. Matheson I and Skajaeraasen J. (1983) Milk concentrations of
     flupenthixol, nortriptyline and zuclopenthixol. *European Journal
     of Clinical Pharmacology*. **35**: 217–20.

81. Aaes-Jorgensen T, Bjorndal F and Bartels U. (1986) Zuclopen-
     thixol levels in serum and breast milk. *Psychopharmacology*. **90**:
     417–18.

82. Polatti F. (1982) Sulpiride isomers and milk secretion in the
     puerperium. *Clinical and Experimental Obstetrics and Gynecology*.
     9: 144–7.

83. Knowles JA. (1965) Excretion of drugs in milk: A review. *Journal
     of Pediatrics*. **66**: 1068–82.

84. Takyi BE. Excretion of drugs in human milk. *Journal of Hospital
     Pharmacy*. **28**: 317–26.

85. Matrangan A. (1971) Drugs excreted in breast milk. *Utah Digest*.
     (Jan) p13. Quoted in O'Brien TE. (1974) Excretion of drugs in
     human milk. *American Journal of Hospital Psychiatry*. **31**: 844–54.

86. Vorherr H. (1974) Drug excretion in breast milk. *Postgraduate
     Medicine*. **56**: 97–104.

87. Sovner R and Orsulak PJ. (1979) Excretion of imipramine and

desipramine in breast milk. *American Journal of Psychiatry.* **136**: 849–50.

88. Erickson SH, Smith GH and Heidrich F. (1979) Tricyclics and breast feeding. *American Journal of Psychiatry.* **136**: 1483.

89. Brixen-Rasmussen L, Halgrener J and Jorgensen A. (1982) Amitriptyline and nortriptyline excretion in breast milk. *Psychopharmacology.* **76**: 94–5.

90. Bader TF and Newman K. (1980) Amitriptyline in human breast milk and the nursing infant's serum. *American Journal of Psychiatry.* **137**: 855–6.

91. Wisner KL and Perel JM. (1991) Serum nortriptyline levels in nursing mothers and their infants. *American Journal of Psychiatry.* **148**: 1234–6.

92. Stancer HC and Reed KL. (1986) Desipramine and 2-hydroxydesipramine in human breast milk and the nursing infant's serum. *American Journal of Psychiatry.* **143**: 1597–1600.

93. Rees JA, Glass RC and Sporne GA. (1976) Serum and breast milk concentrations of dothiepin. *Practitioner.* **217**: 686.

94. Ilett KF, Lebedevs RE, Wojnar-Horton RE, *et al.* (1993) The excretion of dothiepin and its primary metabolites in breast milk. *British Journal of Clinical Pharmacology.* **33**: 635–9.

95. Misri S and Sivertz K. (1991) Tricyclic drugs in pregnancy and lactation: A preliminary report. *International Journal of Psychiatry in Medicine.* **2**: 157–71.

96. Buist A, Norman TR and Dennerstein L. (1993) Mianserin in breast milk. *British Journal of Clinical Pharmacology.* **36**: 133–4.

97. *ABPI Data Sheet Compendium 1991–1992.* Datapharm, London, 298.

98. Lloyd AH. (1977) Practical considerations in the use of maprotiline (Ludiomil) in general practice. *Journal of International Medical Research.* **5**(suppl 4): 122–38.

99. Gelenberg AJ. (1979) Amoxapine, a new antidepressant appears in human milk. *Journal of Nervous and Mental Disease.* **167**: 635–6.

100. Rowan JJ. (1976) Excretion of drugs in milk. *Pharmaceutical Journal.* **217**: 184–5.

101. Pons G, Schoerlin MP, Tam YK, *et al.* (1990) Moclobemide excretion in breast milk. *British Journal of Clinical Pharmacology.* **29**: 27–31.

102. Isenberg KE. (1990) Excretion of fluoxetine in breast milk. *Journal of Clinical Psychiatry.* **51**: 169.

103. Burch KJ and Wells BG. (1992) Fluoxetine/norfluoxetine concentrations in human milk. *Pediatrics.* **89**: 676–7.

104. Verbeeck RK, Ross SG and McKenna EA. (1986) Excretion of trazodone in breast milk. *British Journal of Clinical Pharmacology.* **22**: 367–70.

105. Andersen LW, Qvist T, Hertz J, *et al.* (1987) Concentrations of thiopentone in mature breast milk and colostrum following an induction dose. *Acta Anaesthesiologica Scandinavica.* **31**: 30–2.

106. Pena C, Medina JH, Piva M, *et al.* (1991) Naturally occurring benzodiazepines in human milk. *Biochemical and Biophysical Research Communications.* **175**: 1042–50.

107. Kanto JH. (1982) Use of benzodiazepines during pregnancy, labour and lactation. *Drugs.* **23**: 354–80.

108. Wesson DR, Camber S, Harkey M, *et al.* (1985) Diazepam and desmethyldiazepam in breast milk. *Journal of Psychoactive Drugs.* **17**: 55–6.

109. Anderson PO and McGuire GG. (1990) Neonatal alprazolam withdrawal – possible effects of breast feeding. *Drug Intelligence and Clinical Pharmacy.* **23**: 614.

110. Wretlind M. (1987) Excretion of oxazepam in breast milk. *European Journal of Clinical Pharmacology.* **33**: 209–10.

111. Whitelaw AGL, Cummings AJ and McFadyen IR. (1981) Effect of maternal lorazepam on the neonate. *British Medical Journal.* **282**: 1106–8.

112. Summerfield RJ and Nielsen MS. (1985) Excretion of lorazepam into breast milk. *British Journal of Anaesthetics.* **57**: 1042–3.

113. Dusci LJ, Good SM, Hall RW, *et al.* (1990) Excretion of diazepam and its metabolites in human milk during withdrawal from high

dose diazepam and oxazepam. *British Journal of Clinical Pharmacology*. **29**: 123–6.

114. Lebedevs TH, Wojnar-Horton RE, Yapp P, *et al.* (1992) Excretion of temazepam in breast milk. *British Journal of Clinical Pharmacology*. **33**: 204–6.

115. Matheson I, Lunde PKM and Bredesen JE. (1990) Midazolam and nitrazepam in the maternity ward: Milk concentrations and clinical effects. *British Journal of Clinical Pharmacology*. **30**: 787–93.

116. Bernstine JB, Meyer AE and Bernstine RL. (1956) Maternal blood and breast milk estimation of chloral hydrate. *Journal of Obstetrics and Gynaecology of the British Empire*. **63**: 228–31.

117. Lacey JH. (1971) Dichloralphenazone and breast milk. *British Medical Journal*. **4**: 684.

118. Kaneko S, Suzuki K, Sato T, *et al.* (1982) The problems of antiepileptic medication in the neonatal period: Is breast feeding advisable? In: (Janz D, Bossi L, Dam M, *et al.* editors.) *Epilepsy, pregnancy and the child*. Raven Press, New York, 343–8.

119. Niebyl JR, Blake DA, Freeman JM, *et al.* (1979) Carbamazepine levels in pregnancy and lactation. *Obstetrics and Gynecology*. **53**: 139–40.

120. Kuhnz W, Jager-Roman E, Rating D, *et al.* (1983) Carbamazepine and carbamazepine-10-11-epoxide during pregnancy and postnatal period in epileptic mothers and their nursed infants. *Paediatric Pharmacology*. **3**: 199–208.

121. Froescher W, Eichelbaum M, Niesen M, *et al.* (1984) Carbamazepine levels in breast milk. *Therapeutic Drug Monitoring*. **6**: 266–71.

122. Frey B, Schubiger G and Musy JP. (1990) Transient cholestatic hepatitis in a neonate associated with carbamazepine exposure during pregnancy and breast feeding. *European Journal of Paediatrics*. **150**: 136–8.

123. Fisher JB, Edgren BE, Mammel MC, *et al.* (1985) Neonatal apnoea associated with maternal clonazepam therapy: A case report. *Obstetrics and Gynecology*. **66**(suppl): 34S–35S.

124. Soderman P and Matheson I. (1987) Clonazepam in breast milk. *European Journal of Paediatrics*. **147**: 212–13.

125. Koup JR, Rose JQ and Cohen ME. (1979) Ethosuxamide pharmacokinetics in a pregnant patient and her newborn. *Epilepsia*. **19**: 535–9.

126. Rane A and Tunell R. (1981) Ethosuxamide in human milk and in plasma of a mother and her nursed infant. *British Journal of Clinical Pharmacology*. **12**: 855–8.

127. Kuhnz W, Koch S, Jakob S, *et al*. (1984) Ethosuxamide in epileptic women during pregnancy and lactation period. *British Journal of Clinical Pharmacology*. **18**: 671–7.

128. Kaneko S, Sato T and Suzuki K. (1979) The levels of anticonvulsants in breast milk. *British Journal of Clinical Pharmacology*. **7**: 624–7.

129. Steen B, Rane A, Lonnerholm G, *et al*. (1982) Phenytoin excretion in human breast milk and plasma levels in nursed infants. *Therapeutic Drug Monitoring*. **4**: 331–4.

130. Finch E and Lorber J. (1954) Methaemoglobinaemia in the newborn. *Journal of Obstetrics and Gynaecology of the British Empire*. **61**: 833–4.

131. Nau H, Rating D, Hauser I, *et al*. (1980) Placental transfer and pharmacokinetics of primidone and its metabolites in neonates and infants of epileptic mothers. *European Journal of Clinical Pharmacology*. **18**: 31–41.

132. Granstrom M-L, Bardy AH and Hiilesmaa VK. (1982) Prolonged feeding difficulties in infants of primidone mothers during the neonatal period. In: (Janz D, Bossi L, Dam M, *et al*. editors.) *Epilepsy, pregnancy and the child*. Raven Press, New York, 357–8.

133. Knott C, Reynolds F and Clayden G. (1987) Infantile spasms on weaning from breast milk containing anticonvulsants. *Lancet*. **ii**: 272–3.

134. Nau H, Rating D, Koch S, *et al*. (1981) Valproic acid and its metabolites: Placental transfer, neonatal pharmacokinetics, transfer via mothers milk and clinical status in neonates of epileptic mothers. *Journal of Pharmacology and Experimental Therapeutics*. **219**: 768–77.

135. Philbert A, Pedersen B and Dam M. (1984) Concentration of valproate during pregnancy, in the newborn and in breast milk. *Acta Neurologica Scandinavica.* **72**: 460–3.

136. Schou M and Amdisen A. (1973) Lithium ingestion by children breast fed by women on lithium treatment. *British Medical Journal.* **ii**: 138.

137. Sykes PA and Quarrie J. (1976) Lithium carbonate and breast feeding. *British Medical Journal.* **ii**: 1299.

138. Tunnesen WW and Hertz CG. (1972) Toxic effects of lithium in newborn infants: A commentary. *Journal of Pediatrics.* **81**: 804–7.

139. Wilbanks GD, Bressler B, Peete CH, *et al.* (1970) Toxic effects of lithium carbonate in a mother and new born infant. *JAMA.* **213**: 865–7.

140. Skausig OB and Schou M. (1977) Diegivning under lithium-behandling. *Ugeskrift for Laeger.* **139**: 400–1.

141. Andersen HJ. (1983) Excretion of verapamil in human milk. *European Journal of Clinical Pharmacology.* **25**: 279–80.

142. Inoue H, Unno N, Ou M-C, *et al.* (1984) Level of verapamil in human milk. *European Journal of Clinical Pharmacology.* **26**: 657–8.

143. Miller MR, Withers R, Bhamra R, *et al.* (1986) Verapamil and breast feeding. *European Journal of Clinical Pharmacology.* **30**: 125–6.

144. Anderson P, Bondesson U, Mattiasson I, *et al.* (1987) Verapamil and norverapamil in plasma and breast milk. *European Journal of Clinical Pharmacology.* **31**: 625–7.

145. Bauer JH, Pape B, Zajicek J, *et al.* (1979) Propranolol in human plasma and breast milk. *American Journal of Cardiology.* **43**: 860–2.

146. Schimmel MS, Eidelman AJ, Wilschanski MA, *et al.* (1989) Toxic effects of atenolol consumed during breast feeding. *Journal of Pediatrics.* **114**: 476–8.

147. Koetsawang S. (1987) The effects of contraceptive methods on the quality and quantity of breast milk. *International Journal of Gynaecology and Obstetrics.* **25**(suppl): 115–27.

148. Laukaran VH. (1987) The effects of contraceptive use on the initiation and duration of lactation. *International Journal of Gynaecology and Obstetrics*. **25**(suppl): 129–42.

149. McCann MF, Moggia AV, Higgins JE, *et al.* (1989) The effects of a progesterone-only oral contraceptive on breast feeding. *Contraception*. **40**: 635–48.

150. Nilsson S, Nygren K-G and Johanssen EDB. (1978) Transfer of oestradiol to human milk. *American Journal of Obstetrics and Gynecology*. **132**: 653–7.

151. Nilsson S and Nygren K-G. (1979) Transfer of contraceptive steroids to human milk. *Research in Reproduction*. **1**: 1–2.

152. Harlap S. (1987) Exposure to contraceptive hormones through breast milk. *International Journal of Gynaecology and Obstetrics*. **25**(suppl): 47–55.

153. Curtis EM. (1964) Oral contraceptive feminisation of a normal male infant. *Obstetrics and Gynecology*. **23**: 295–6.

154. Madhapaveddi R and Ramachandran P. (1985) Side effects of oral contraceptive use in lactating women. *Contraception*. **32**: 437–53.

155. Nilsson S, Melbin T, Hofvander Y, *et al.* (1986) Long term follow up of children breast fed by mothers on oral contraceptives. *Contraception*. **34**: 443–57.

156. Dalton K. (1985) Progesterone prophylaxis used successfully in postnatal depression. *Practitioner*. **229**: 507–8.

157. Greene R and Dalton K. (1953) The premenstrual syndrome. *British Medical Journal*. **ii**: 1007–14.

158. Sato T and Suzuki Y. (1979) Presence of triiodothyronine, no detectable thyroxine and reverse triiodothyronine in human milk. *Endocrinologica Japonica*. **26**: 507–13.

159. Oberkotter LV and Hahn HB. (1983) Thyroid function and human breast milk. *American Journal of Diseases of Children*. **137**: 1131.

160. Oberkotter LV. (1989) Analysis of human milk concentrations of 3, 5, 3, triiodo-L-thyronine: Correlation with serum levels in lactating women. *Journal of Chromatography*. **487**: 445–8.

161. Cooper DS. (1987) Antithyroid drugs: To breast feed or not to breast feed. *American Journal of Obstetrics and Gynecology.* **157**: 234–5.

162. Lamberg B-A, Ikonen E, Osterlund K, *et al.* (1984) Antithyroid treatment of maternal hypothyroidism during lactation. *Clinical Endocrinology.* **21**: 81–7.

163. Rylance GW, Woods CG, Donnelly MC, *et al.* (1987) Carbimazole and breast feeding. *Lancet.* **i**: 928.

164. Momotani N, Yamashita R, Yoshimoto M, *et al.* (1989) Recovery from foetal hypothyroidism: Evidence for the safety of breast feeding on propylthiouracil. *Clinical Endocrinology.* **31**: 591–5.

Further Reading

Brockington IF and Kumar R. (1982) Drug addiction and psychotropic drug treatment during pregnancy and lactation. In: *Motherhood and mental illness.* Academic Press, London, 239–55.

Kochenour NK and Emery MG. (1981) Drugs in lactating women. *Obstetric and Gynaecology Annual.* **10**: 107–26.

Anderson PO. (1991) Drug use during breast feeding. *Clinical Pharmacy.* **10**: 594–624.

Wilson JT, Brown RD, Cherek DR, *et al.* (1980) Drug excretion in human breast milk. *Clinical Pharmacokinetics.* **5**: 1–66.

Reisner SH, Eisenberg NH, Stahl B, *et al.* (1983) Maternal medications and breast feeding. *Developmental Pharmacology and Therapeutics.* **6**: 285–304.

9   Fathers

We have seen in preceding chapters how childbirth, a 'happy event', can in some cases, have profound negative implications for the mother's mental health during pregnancy and, most of all, during the puerperium. In many research studies, the quality of the relationship with the partner has been found to have a significant part to play in the causation of the mother's illness. However, men as well as women have complicated and variable reactions to the birth of a child, and there is growing interest in the interaction of the couple in the transition to parenthood[1-3]. The impact of puerperal illness in the mother may also have profound effects on the mental health of her partner[4].

The decision to have a child is not always a mutual one. One survey found that 25% of pregnancies were unplanned, and that a further 8% were largely as a result of the mother's decision alone[5].

The Father's Role During Pregnancy

Preparation for parenthood is important for fathers as well as mothers. The emphasis of current antenatal teaching for fathers often seems to be on the factual aspects of labour, familiarizing them with procedures and equipment, and encouraging them to be present at the birth. Few classes seem to give fathers time to express their own feelings. Relatively few fathers appear to attend all antenatal education classes, and even less attend routine antenatal appointments. Perhaps if there were evening sessions, or if there were a crèche provided, this would become more usual.

The majority of women report increased dependency needs during pregnancy[1,5,6]. It seems that most partners can respond by increasing their nurturing behaviour, but rarely enough to satisfy the pregnant mother. The partner's need for nurturance may also increase towards the end of pregnancy, and there are indications that the pregnant mother becomes more preoccupied, and is less able to give affection to her partner as pregnancy progresses. There may also be a change in dominance patterns, particularly in 'wife-dominated' relationships[1]. First-time parents seem to express higher levels of affection to each other throughout pregnancy.

Most fathers become aware of their increased financial and practical responsibility towards the family, particularly when the woman's income has been a substantial part of the family budget. This anxiety may lead to extra commitments at work, either in overtime, or striving for promotion, so that he is less available to provide the emotional support needed. Anxiety measured by self-report scales in first-time expectant fathers has, surprisingly, been found to be lower than the population norm, and lower than that of fathers whose partners were not pregnant. This has been interpreted as a conscious denial of anxiety in an attempt to project strength and reliability in the face of the mother's increasing dependency[7]. However, there may also be an aspect of satisfaction at the proof of fertility, or at the increasing dominance of the male role within the partnership as the pregnancy progresses.

The presence of depressive symptoms in either partner has been examined. Nearly 40% of couples had one partner who was depressed in late pregnancy; in 37% of these, it was the husband with symptoms. It was rare for both partners to experience depressed mood simultaneously[8].

Thirty-two per cent of a group of men reported an increase in anxiety during their partners' pregnancies, compared with 61% of the pregnant mothers. The men attributed their anxiety largely to concerns about whether the arrival of a baby would damage the marital relationship[9]. These fears appear to be well founded. In one study, many couples showed an increased closeness within the relationship, but at least 10% had significantly weakened marriages by 12 months' postpartum, with younger couples and marriages of shorter duration more at risk[3]. Another author has found that up to 70% of husbands felt that they had drifted apart from their spouses in certain ways during the first postnatal year[10].

The concept of 'couvade', ritualized in many primitive

societies, is a process whereby the father experiences pain or discomfort in parallel with the pregnant or labouring woman. This was thought to originate in attempts to divert evil influences from the pregnancy, and also perhaps to confirm the father's true paternity. It seems to persist to the present day in western society in the form of increased minor somatic symptoms in fathers. This can be detected as early as three months into the pregnancy, and persists until after the birth. The symptoms are generally mild and non-specific and include fatigue, nausea, backache and abdominal pain[11]. An interesting finding is that many men put on weight when their partners are pregnant. Physical symptoms seem to be less in those men who are more emotionally involved with the pregnancy.

The Father's Role During Labour

Fathers are generally present at the birth of the child, and their absence is often taken to be due to a lack of involvement. Most feel positive about the experience, even if they have had prior doubts about their ability to cope; almost all say that they would choose to be present at a subsequent delivery.

The father's role in the delivery room is often not clearly defined. He is there to offer 'support' to his partner, but without clear directions about how to do so. Fathers often seem to feel superfluous in the female-dominated situation, and may defend themselves against their own anxiety by becoming interested in the technological equipment, or aligning themselves with male doctors. Many see their role as mediators between the woman in labour and the staff, interpreting procedures, and describing what is happening.

The moment of birth is an emotional one for both parents, and often produces a spontaneous display of affection between them. It is common for fathers not to feel immediate attachment for their newborn child, but this does not mean that they will be uncommitted parents in the future. There is evidence that men interact rather more with male infants at birth[2].

The Father's Role Postpartum

The most obvious change postpartum is that a partnership with an egalitarian basis resolves itself into 'mother and father' with greater differentiation of roles. Many women embark on a pregnancy with the expectation that the father will share in child care, only to be disappointed about the actual degree of his practical commitment. Even when the father takes leave from work after the birth, child care is seen largely as the mother's role. On his return to work he may indeed be less involved in household practicalities because the mother is at home all day. With regard to involvement with the child, one study found that 40% of fathers had never or rarely changed a nappy by the time the baby was one year old, and that fewer had ever bathed the child[5]. Uninvolved men were generally those whose work commitments prevented them from being helpful, and those who continued to have social interests and hobbies apart from the family, and saw no reason to modify this after the birth. In some cases, this seems to be an active avoidance of commitment to the mother and child as a result of the father's own feelings of distress.

Much has been written in psychoanalytical literature about men's reactions to their first child in particular. The baby is interpreted as a rival for the mother's affection, reawakening earlier conflicts from his own childhood. Oedipal conflicts are those in which the male child has hateful fantasies towards his father, wishing to have his mother all to himself. These may be reawakened by the birth of a child when the partner becomes 'mother', preoccupied with the needs of another, and unable to give him the affection he needs. Studies of men's needs for nurturance have found that less than half the fathers expressed satisfaction with the wife's ability to give it at one month postpartum; the proportion fell to 40% by six months[1]. This feeling of 'exclusion' from the closeness of mother and child is undoubtedly exacerbated by the normal decrease in libido experienced by women in late pregnancy and the first post-partum year[12].

If he himself has had a distant or inadequate father, he may fear being an inadequate parent himself, and his feelings towards his own child may highlight deficiencies in his own experience of parenting, leading to ambivalence towards his family of origin. It has in fact been demonstrated that men with a poor relationship with their children also have poor relationships with their own fathers[13]. The birth may also reactivate feelings of rage and jealousy felt at the birth of a younger sibling.

Mental Illness in Fathers

About one-third of fathers experience some mood disorder in the early postpartum months, relating this to the changes within the marriage. At three months, these men were less involved with the baby, both emotionally and practically, but by 12 months, they were more involved than a control group. The mood changes appeared to be mild, relatively short-lived, and did not require treatment[7].

A recent study has identified 9% of fathers as 'cases' of depression at six weeks postpartum, and 5.4% at six months. The incidence in mothers was 27.5% and 25.7% at the same intervals. Fathers were significantly more likely to be depressed if their partners were too[14].

There are isolated accounts of severe mental illness occurring in fathers at the time of their partner's pregnancy or soon after delivery[15-17]. Whether the cause is specifically related to pregnancy, whether the pregnancy is simply a life event giving rise to a non-specific stress, or whether the two are simply coincidental, is unclear.

Partners of Women with Puerperal Mental Illness

It is not surprising that the partners of women who become mentally ill after childbirth should be disturbed themselves. In the case of puerperal psychosis, where the illness is severe, sudden in onset, and distressing in character, psychological distress in the partner is almost inevitable.

One recent study found that 42% of the partners of women admitted to a mother and baby unit had marked psychiatric morbidity, compared with only 4% of controls[4]. In another, 50% of partners had a psychiatric diagnosis, although most of the disorders diagnosed were mild and transient[18]. In many of these men there was a previous personal history of psychiatric illness.

This finding has important implications for the treatment of women with puerperal psychiatric disorder. Not only may the mother's recovery be delayed, but there are also indications that the father's illness may have a detrimental effect on the emotional development of the child[19,20]. It goes without saying that fathers should be given as much information as possible about mothers' illnesses, and should be intimately involved in treatment plans. However, a significant number may also need counselling and treatment in their own right before they are able to give adequate support to their partners and families.

References

1. Scott-Heyes G. (1983) Marital adaptation during pregnancy and after childbirth. *Journal of Reproductive and Infant Psychology.* **1**: 18–28.

2. Woollett EA, White DG and Lyons ML. (1982) Observations on fathers at birth. In: (Beail N and McGuire J editors.) *Fathers: Psychological perspectives.* Junction Books, London, 71–91.

3. Moss P, Bolland G, Foxman R, *et al.* (1986) Marital relations during the transition to parenthood. *Journal of Reproductive and Infant Psychology.* **4**: 57–67.

4. Harvey I and McGrath G. (1988) Psychiatric morbidity in spouses of women admitted to a mother and baby unit. *British Journal of Psychiatry.* **152**: 506–10.

5. Nicolson P. (1990) A brief report of women's expectations of men's behaviour in the transition to parenthood. *Counselling Psychology Quarterly.* **3**: 353–61.

6. Wenner N, Cohen MB, Weigert EV, *et al.* (1969) Emotional problems of pregnancy. *Psychiatry.* **39**: 389–410.

7. Teichman Y and Lahav Y. (1987) Expectant fathers: Emotional reactions, physical symptoms and coping styles. *British Journal of Medical Psychology.* **60**: 225–32.

8. Raskin VD, Richman JA and Gaines C. (1990) Patterns of depressive symptoms in expectant and new parents. *American Journal of Psychiatry.* **147**: 658–60.

9. Condon JT. (1987) Psychological and physical symptoms during pregnancy: A comparison of male and female expectant parents. *Journal of Reproductive and Infant Psychology.* **5**: 207–13.

10. Lewis C. (1986) *Becoming a father.* Open University Press, Milton Keynes.

11. Shereshevsky PM and Yarrow LJ. (1974) *Psychological aspects of a first pregnancy and early postnatal adaptation.* Raven Press, New York.

12. Alder EM, Cook A, Davidson D, *et al.* (1986) Hormones, mood and sexuality and lactating women. *British Journal of Psychiatry.* **148**: 74–9.

13. Nettelbladt P, Uddenberg N and Englesson I. (1980) Father/child relationship: Background factors in the father. *Acta Psychiatrica Scandinavica.* **61**: 29–42.

14. Ballard C, Davis R and Dean C. (1994) Postnatal depression in mothers and fathers. In: *Recent advances in childbearing and mental health.* Abstracts of the 6th International Conference of the Marcé Society. *British Journal of Psychiatry.* **164**: 782–8.

15. Asch SS and Rubin LJ. (1974) Postpartum reactions: Some unrecognised variations. *American Journal of Psychiatry.* **131**: 870–4.

16. Freeman T. (1951) Pregnancy as a precipitant of mental illness in men. *British Journal of Medical Psychology.* **24**: 49–54.

17. Wainwright WH. (1966) Fatherhood as a precipitant of mental illness. *American Journal of Psychiatry.* **123**: 40–4.

18. Lovestone S and Kumar R. (1993) Postnatal psychiatric illness: The impact on partners. *British Journal of Psychiatry.* **163**: 210–16.

19. Murray L, Cooper PJ and Stein A. (1991) Postnatal depression and infant development. *British Medical Journal.* **309**: 978–9.

20. Caplan HL, Coghill SR, Alexandra H, *et al.* (1989) Maternal depression and the emotional development of the child. *British Journal of Medical Psychology.* **154**: 818–22.

Further Reading

Beail N and McGuire J, editors. (1982) *Fathers: Psychological perspectives.* Junction Books, London.

Lewis C and O'Brien M, editors. (1987) *Reassessing fatherhood.* Sage, London.

Niven CA. (1992) *Psychological care for families*. Butterworth Heinemann, Oxford.

Raphael-Leff J. (1991) *Psychological processes of childbearing*. Chapman & Hall, London.

Robson B and Mandel D. (1985) Marital adjustment and fatherhood. *Canadian Journal of Psychiatry*. **30**: 169–72.

10   Service Provision

Improvement of Existing Services

Some of the alterations to antenatal and postnatal services that might help to prevent or ameliorate emotional distress for mothers have been touched on briefly in other chapters. Above all, what seems to be needed is a change in orientation and emphasis from the largely physical model of pregnancy and childbirth to the appreciation of the event primarily as an emotional experience, set in the wider context of the mother's psychosocial environment.

The birth of a first child, in particular, forms a 'rite of passage' from young adulthood to maturity for both parents. It is exciting and challenging, but also loaded with uncertainty and anxiety. It represents a loss of freedom and of self-interest, as well as a gain. Never again will the couple be so carefree; the responsibility of a child is awesome and appears interminable as well as rewarding and fulfilling. Becoming a parent also leads to identification with their own parents, and a reawakening of childhood experiences, both good and bad. It changes the social, economic and emotional roles of both partners.

We have seen how those mothers with marital difficulties or inadequate community support are more vulnerable to depression both before and after the birth. We can therefore deduce that provision of a confiding relationship and attention to the social setting of the mother can be preventative. This is often a function of the obstetric social worker. However, a referral to social workers is often only made for women with the most chaotic life-style, and may be felt by the woman herself to be a criticism of her mothering ability. She may also be unwilling to have contact with social workers because of fears about her children being taken into care.

The Midwife's Role

The booking interview is already time-consuming for the midwife, but it is the mother's first contact with the obstetric service. Because of the emotional investment the mother brings to the first interview, she will probably relate better to the midwife she first encounters than to others. Perhaps a later interview with the same midwife could explore some of the wider family dynamics, such as support from the partner, the family of origin, or friends and neighbours. This interview could also be the opportunity to express feelings about the pregnancy, not just anxieties about its normality, but how welcome it is at this particular time in this particular woman's life, and what adjustments she will need to make.

Later in the pregnancy, further exploration could be made of the mother's expectations of labour, and any particular fears she may have. She may also benefit from forward planning about suitable help in the home postpartum.

We also know that mothers appreciate continuity of care from the professionals attending them. Although some attempts have been made to provide more continuity, perhaps more could be done. In line with the recent provision of mental health teams established on a geographical basis, perhaps mothers could be allocated to an obstetric team, leading to involvement with a smaller number of personnel, and easier contact with other mothers in the same area due to have their babies at about the same time.

The Antenatal Teacher's Role

Antenatal classes, as we have seen, are variable in quality and content, tend to include more middle-class than working-class women, and few men. The educators may be midwives, health visitors, physiotherapists or other paramedicals with their own individual orientation about what and how to teach.

Various suggestions have been made about how to improve such teaching. One authority in South Africa has suggested a childbirth education diploma, to be recognized as a postgraduate qualification[1]. The objectives were for training to be multidisciplinary, drawing on both biological and social sciences. It was based on the assumption that preparation for parenthood involves a holistic view of pregnancy, birth, and early parenthood, and that such preparation should be directed towards couples or families rather than only mothers. Apart from basic knowledge of anatomy, physiology and obstetrics, the objectives included:

- being able to prepare parents for the physical, emotional and behavioural aspects of becoming a parent

- having an adequate knowledge of the impact of the birth of a baby on family life, both nuclear and extended

- having an understanding of variations in the psychological and behavioural approaches to childbirth amongst parents from different ethnic or cultural backgrounds

- being able to counsel parents whose pregnancies end in still birth or miscarriage

- being able to offer basic counselling to parents as well as to recognize when their skills are inadequate and when referral is needed

- being conversant with emotional problems arising during or after the pregnancy, eg the 'blues', postnatal depression and puerperal psychosis.

How to Acquire the Skills?

Some professional carers have their own anxieties about becoming involved with their clients on a more emotional level. They fear opening the 'Pandora's box' of feelings because they have neither the skills nor the time to deal with them.

A suggestion about suitable training requirements has come from authorities in Holland, who have proposed that education in the psychosocial, psychosomatic and psychosexual aspects of obstetrics and gynaecology should be in terms of knowledge, attitudes and skills[2]. Under the heading of attitudes, they include:

- insight into the relationships of the patient (partner, family, work, culture) and their influence on her well-being, physical and psychological functioning

- insight into the management of one's own emotions and psychosocial thinking in relation to the patient's problems

- insight into the handling of one's own limitations and failures

- understanding the changing social norms and values of society pertaining to sexuality, reproduction and sex roles.

They felt that the teaching of attitudes was largely by example from the teaching staff, but should include audiovisual material and group experience. Skills could be taught by seminar, and by practice (eg as a co-therapist) and should include:

- acquisition of communication skills (listening as well as speaking)

- the ability to take a psychosocial and sexual history

- the ability to detect and evaluate concealed or overt psychological, psychosocial and sexual problems.

These authors conclude that a team approach is most appropriate, with specifically interested staff supported by social workers, psychologists and psychiatrists.

It would be ideal if these principles could be included in current midwifery and health visitor training. Alternatively, they could form the basis of a specialist diploma.

Other Forms of Training

The Marcé Society is an international association of psychiatrists, psychologists, midwives and other interested professionals who are concerned with the understanding, prevention and treatment of mental illness related to childbearing. Similarly, the Society for Reproductive and Infant Psychology consists of many health professionals who have expertise in this area. Where professionals with a special interest are available, it is important to use their expertise in training courses.

Both of the above societies organize regular meetings in which recent research results are presented, and good examples of service provision are discussed.

Sadly, not all midwifery schools and health visitor training courses have the same access to local professionals who are willing to teach on these topics. As a result, the Marcé Society conducted a market research project on the interest in a 'distance learning' programme on the emotional aspects of childbirth. The response was overwhelmingly favourable, and the programme is currently being written. It will include the topics mentioned above. The course requires the student to be able to recognize both the normal and abnormal emotional responses associated with pregnancy and birth, to acquire the ability to undertake counselling and support, and to know when more specialized help is needed. It can be undertaken at any stage in midwifery or health visitor training, or as part of a refresher course, and would be equally appropriate for community psychiatric nurses, medical students and other interested professionals. The course is equally suitable for students working in isolation, as a study group, or with a tutor.

Psychiatric Services

There are few areas that provide a specialized service for psychologically disturbed mothers. In many cases, the emphasis has been largely on the provision of in-patient facilities for mothers suffering from the severe end of the spectrum of psychiatric disorder. Even fewer areas have access to a truly comprehensive obstetric liaison service[3-5]. It has been shown that admissions for postnatal illness can be reduced in number and in length where there is a specialist obstetric liaison psychiatrist in post. A recent audit of preventative intervention with a 'high-risk' group of pregnant women has also shown that psychiatric intervention in pregnancy can reduce the incidence of PND by one-third, and almost abolish the need for postnatal admission for previously psychotic patients[6]. This audit also showed that there is still a stigma about psychiatric intervention, and there is clearly a case for specially trained and experienced community psychiatric nurses who can provide home-based counselling and continuity of care. Perhaps even more importantly, the presence of a specialist in a health district can encourage and support the expertise of midwives and primary care teams, creating a network of preventative, screening and early treatment options.

Mother and baby units

The idea of admitting babies with their psychiatrically disturbed mothers was pioneered in the 1940s by Dr Tom Main at the Cassel Hospital. This was as a result of much research into the adverse effects on the child of separation from its mother. However, the Cassel only admitted those with neurotic, rather than psychotic, disorders, and the emphasis of treatment was on prolonged admission and psychotherapy.

Other units followed suit, although not without trepidation about the risks of harm to the baby. At one hospital, for example, the mothers were assessed alone on an admission ward until they were judged suitable to care for the baby, and, even then, the supervision was extreme and intrusive. The mother was continuously 'shadowed' by a nurse, and was not allowed to handle her baby during the night. Over the years, experience has shown that the risk of deliberate harm to such babies is low[7], and that mothers recover more quickly and relapse less often when joint admissions are possible[8].

A recent survey showed that only 19% of all health districts in England and Wales have dedicated facilities for mother and baby admissions, and in only just over half of these was there a local consultant with a special interest in obstetric liaison work. Nevertheless, 73% of those replying to the questionnaire thought that such provision was important and a resource priority[9].

The difficulty with these facilities is that they are expensive to staff, and the bed occupancy may be low because of intermittent demand. Regional units do exist, and provide useful tertiary referral centres with excellent standards of care. However, the rehabilitation of mother and baby into their own home is an important part of the treatment plan, and this is more difficult to arrange both in geographical terms, and in the necessary liaison with local primary care facilities, when the mother is far from her own home.

The ideal unit has been described as one which should include day hospital and day nursery services as well as an in-patient unit, so that it can care for older children as well as babies, and for mothers with moderate levels of psychiatric disturbance not requiring admission. Where the catchment area is large, facilities for fathers to stay overnight should also be available. Such a unit could also provide a resource centre and training unit.

Day hospitals

These provide a useful alternative to admission for mothers with only moderately severe illness. The experience in Stoke-on-Trent has shown that mothers benefit from the nursing input, the shared experience of others, and social contacts; the children also receive a great deal of stimulation which they might otherwise lack[10]. However, the success of the service depends on good transport facilities to an urban centre with a high population density and birth rate. It is probably not suitable for a large rural area.

Community care

Many psychiatrically ill women are reluctant to accept in-patient care, often because there are older children at home. An outstandingly successful service in Nottingham has provided care, even for psychotic patients, within their own homes[11]. The criteria for community care were that the woman should live within a 20-minute drive of the hospital, and that there was another responsible adult, usually a family member, living at the patient's home. The input varies from eight hours' continuous nursing care daily, to visits from a community nurse on alternate days.

The service requires the back-up of a mother and baby unit, and an experienced multidisciplinary team. It is not an inexpensive option, although savings can clearly be made in terms of in-patient provision.

Out-patient therapy groups

These can be a relatively inexpensive and useful facility for mothers with neurotic disorders, who have an ability and a wish to examine emotional issues[12,13]. They require the provision of a crèche, so that the mothers can concentrate on themselves, and therapists who are interested in the work and sufficiently experienced to deal with some of the powerful feelings that may surface during the sessions. Because of the need for early intervention, and the high drop-out rate, 'slow-open' groups are probably most suitable, with mothers leaving or joining at natural breaks in the series of sessions. Unlike other psychotherapy groups, the mothers may need a time after each session to 'wind down' before resuming care of the children. Transport is also needed if the group is in a sparsely populated area.

Individual therapy
This is not easy to obtain within the National Health Service. In many cases, there will be a delay between referral and acceptance, and the therapy offered may be brief; a course of 12 weekly sessions is often all that is available. Private psychotherapy is often too expensive to contemplate. However, in many areas there are local counselling services, branches of the Westminster Pastoral Foundation, and MIND, where counselling and therapy is available at low or no cost.

The LIFE organization is supportive to single mothers, and rape crisis centres are often able to offer counselling for the late effects of sexual abuse. Marital and psychosexual counselling is available from most branches of RELATE.

Self-help groups
These can be set up by professionals or by recovered women, but it is important for them to have an interested professional to turn to if they feel that more intensive help is needed. One woman writes of her experience in such a group.

> 'At the meetings we try to create an atmosphere where it's OK to talk about problems, and some of us who are or have been depressed have found that we can admit to thoughts, feelings and experiences we could not discuss with husbands, friends or even doctors. It's a relief to find that you're not alone in having panic attacks, or being unable to trust your nearest and dearest, or having to drag yourself out of bed in the mornings. . . . It's encouraging to see that other women have recovered and to find that fellow-sufferers can be likeable people – it helps you believe that you might still be likeable too.'[14]

Individual befriending
This is often appropriate for the depressed mother who finds social contact difficult. The National Childbirth Trust have postnatal counsellors who can support depressed women in their own homes, and the Association for Postnatal Illness has a telephone support line through which mothers can be put in touch with local ex-sufferers.

Early identification of postnatal illness

Clearly, picking up the early signs of emotional distress can lead to intervention at a stage when the problems can be prevented from escalating. The postnatal examination is an ideal opportunity, not only to check the physical recovery from the birth, but also the mother's emotional adjustment.

One district in Buckinghamshire is running a pilot study in which all newly delivered mothers are screened by the health visitor, using the Edinburgh Postnatal Depression Scale, at about five weeks postpartum. Those with high scores are to be given increased health visitor support, and will have the test repeated two weeks later. If the score is persistently high, the health visitor offers up to eight regular weekly counselling sessions, including the father in at least one of these. A further assessment at the end of the sessions indicates whether referral for further treatment is needed. This of course implies that the health visitors are willing and able to carry out the programme, that suitable training in counselling techniques is available, and that there is sufficient back-up from interested family doctors and psychiatric staff.

Preventative intervention

The identification of vulnerable women at an early stage of the pregnancy allows for intervention before the possible onset of postnatal problems. It has been shown that those women receiving counselling from health visitors during the pregnancy have a lower incidence of morbidity in the postnatal period compared with equally vulnerable women who were not given this experience[15].

The history of previous psychiatric illness in the woman or her first degree relatives is probably the most significant vulnerability factor, and this is generally noted at the booking clinic. However, there are other important factors, such as the woman's own experience of mothering, and her satisfaction with the relationship with the partner, which are probably not recorded. It would be helpful to have a brief questionnaire on these issues for patients to complete during the first clinic appointment. It would need to be brief, quick to complete, and simple for midwives to score, so that an overall and more accurate measure of vulnerability can be gained.

For this screening to be effective, intervention has to be available. This could be provided by health visitors, or better still, by a multidisciplinary team including community psychiatric nurses (CPN), who could provide counselling either on an individual or a group basis. One such CPN has written of her experience[16], making several important points.

- The CPN becomes involved in antenatal education, talking about postnatal depression. This allows the mothers to get to know her and her role at an early stage.

- Fathers, who are probably those best placed to detect early signs of illness, are also given this information.

- The CPN accepts referrals directly from midwives and health visitors – a 'short cut' compared with the traditional contact via family doctor and consultant.

- The CPN also conducts postnatal support groups, so that there is continuity of care.

Conclusions

The problem of perinatal emotional disorder in all its degrees of severity is an important issue, in both social and economic terms. Discussions with the Department of Health in 1985 led to the formation of a working party on the subject. The recent report from this body[17] has noted the 'significant unmet need' of women with puerperal mental disorders, and the inequality of service provision in different areas. The authors conclude that the skills needed are best acquired and carried out by a specialist consultant-led scheme, including community psychiatric nurses, with close links to primary care. The team should provide a district or supra-district service.

To this end, they suggest:

- greater emphasis on the subject in undergraduate medical training

- inclusion of similar teaching during vocational training for family doctors

- greater emphasis on the subject in postgraduate psychiatric training

- inclusion of teaching on the subject as part of continuing medical education

- inclusion of these topics in the training of health visitors, midwives, community psychiatric nurses and social workers.

The report goes on to make recommendations about service provision, emphasizing the need for care to be 'rapid, appropriate, accessible and effective' and provided by health professionals who 'possess the appropriate skills, experiences and resources'.

However, the reality is that, sadly, there is still a stigma attached to being a psychiatric patient, and there are inadequate numbers of interested and experienced psychiatrists currently working in this field.

We should, therefore, be using these specialists to spread their expertise by teaching and encouraging those who are already in contact with pregnant and postnatal women to use their existing skills more widely and to greater effect. We should be offering midwives, health visitors and general practitioners suitable information and training in the prevention and early detection of emotional disorders associated with pregnancy, childbirth and the first postnatal year. The Marcé Society distance learning project and this book are the first steps in a wider educational initiative.

The *Health of the Nation* document[18] sets out three primary targets:

- to improve significantly the health and social functioning of mentally ill people

- to reduce the overall suicide rate by at least 15% by the year 2000

- to reduce the suicide rate of severely mentally ill people by at least 33% by the year 2000.

It suggests that all staff – primary health care teams, social workers, day and home care staff, midwives, casualty staff and hospital and community doctors and nurses – should have better training in the recognition and treatment of mental illness. The document singles out postnatal mental illness as one of the crucial areas where the development of these skills is particularly beneficial.

That the interest and enthusiasm is there is not in doubt. The number of people attending seminars and lectures on the subject clearly shows the thirst for knowledge. Many midwives and other health professionals write to the Marcé Society for further sources of information to help them with educational projects or simply to help them deal sensitively with their patients.

A recent paper on the wider issues of mental health[19] states:

'A comprehensive mental health service must be based above all on prevention. It must also provide treatment for those who have escaped the preventive net. ... Prevention must depend first and foremost on the availability of appropriate help for those who care for children – especially mothers of babies.'

It goes on to assert that:

'Ideally placed to be the front-line troops are the Health Visitors. If each had similar support from a therapeutic caseworker – who should be prepared to take over any unduly difficult case – Health Visitors in the course of their ordinary duties could enable many healthy mothers to get things right with their babies from the start, and thus avoid the problems for which they might otherwise need (but probably fail to receive) more specialised treatment.'

An equally cogent case can be argued for the midwife and obstetrician, who are the most important monitors of maternal mental, as well as physical, health during pregnancy and immediately after delivery.

Postscript

There are many other important issues related to the mental health of women which this book has not attempted to cover –

miscarriage, perinatal bereavement, infertility, the new fertility technology, the effect of maternal psychiatric illness on the child and family – to name but a few. The author's intention was to create a condensation of very basic facts about prenatal and postnatal mental health in the hope that it will act as a springboard for all those interested in being more involved in this complex but rewarding subject.

References

1. Chalmers BE and Hofmeyr GF. (1989) The gestation of a child-birth diploma. *Journal of Psychosomatic Obstetrics and Gynaecology.* **10**: 179–87.

2. Van Hall EV, Bos G, van der Lugt B, *et al.* (1982) A proposal for training requirements concerning the psychosomatic, psychosocial and psychosexual aspects of the speciality obstetrics and gynaecology. *Journal of Psychosomatic Obstetrics and Gynaecology.* **1**: 91–2.

3. Riley D. (1986) An audit of obstetric liaison psychiatry. *Journal of Reproductive and Infant Psychology.* **4**: 99–115.

4. Appleby L, Fox H, Shaw M, *et al.* (1989) The psychiatrist in the obstetric unit – establishing a liaison service. *British Journal of Psychiatry.* **154**: 510–15.

5. Phillips N and Dennerstein L. (1993) The psychiatrist in an obstetric/gynaecology hospital: Establishing a consultation-liaison service. *Australian and New Zealand Journal of Psychiatry.* **27**: 464–71.

6. Quinton C, Riley D and Cooper S. (1993) Does psychiatric consultation in pregnancy prevent postnatal depression? *Auditorium.* **2**: 58–62.

7. Margison FR. (1990) Infants of mentally ill mothers: The risk of injury and its control. *Journal of Reproductive and Infant Psychology.* **8**: 137–46.

8. Lindsay JSB and Pollard DE. (1978) Mothers and children in hospital. *Australian and New Zealand Journal of Psychiatry.* **12**: 245–53.

9. Prettyman RJ and Friedman T. (1991) Care of women with puerperal psychiatric disorders in England and Wales. *British Medical Journal.* **302**: 1245–6.

10. Cox JL, Gerrard J, Cookson D, *et al.* (1993) Development and audit

of Charles Street Parent and Baby Day Unit, Stoke-on-Trent. *Psychiatric Bulletin.* **17**: 711–13.

11. Oates M. (1988) The development of an integrated community-orientated service for severe postnatal mental illness. In: *Motherhood and mental illness* 2. Wright, London, 133–58.

12. Morris JB. (1987) Group therapy for prolonged postnatal depression. *British Journal of Medical Psychology.* **60**: 279–81.

13. Goulden A and Dorkings E. (1992) A mothers' group in a child guidance clinic. *Psychiatric Bulletin.* **16**: 286–7.

14. Bairstow S. (1986) Coping with postnatal depression. In: Levy L, *Finding our own solutions.* Women in Mind Publications, London, 97–9.

15. Holden JM, Sagovsky R and Cox JL. (1989) Counselling in a general practice setting: A controlled study of health visitor intervention in the treatment of postnatal depression. *British Medical Journal.* **298**: 223–6.

16. Dube R. (1992) Postnatal depression: A community psychiatric nurse's view. *Bulletin of the Marcé Society.* (Autumn): 17–20.

17. Report of the General Psychiatry Section Working Party on Postnatal Mental Illness. (1992) *Psychiatric Bulletin.* **16**: 519–22.

18. Department of Health. (1993) The health of the nation: Key area handbook on mental illness. HMSO, London.

19. Woodmansey AC. (1989) Reversing the vicious spiral: A radical approach to mental health. *British Journal of Clinical and Social Psychiatry.* **6**: 103–6.

11   Resources

Helpful Addresses

Active Birth Centre
55 Dartmouth Park Road, London NW5 1SL
071 267 3006
Runs nationwide courses on natural childbirth. Rents birth pools.

Association of Breastfeeding Mothers
26 Holmshaw Close, London SE26 4TH
081 778 4769
Counselling service and local support groups for mothers.

Association of Chartered Physiotherapists in Obstetrics and Gynaecology
Ruth Hawkes, 1 The Cottages, High Street, North Scarle, Lincoln LN6 9EP
Offers advice about posture, muscle tone and exercise in pregnancy and postpartum.

AIMS (Association for the Improvement of Maternity Services)
c/o Beverley Beech, 21 Iver Lane, Iver, Bucks SL0 9LH
0753 652781
Offers support advice and information about maternity rights and options. Send SAE.

Association for Postnatal Illness (APNI)
25 Jerdan Place, Fulham, London SW6 1BE
071 386 0868
Telephone advice and befriending for PND. Supports research and issues newsletter.

Association for Spina Bifida and Hydrocephalus (ASBAH)
ASBAH House, 42 Park Road, Peterborough PE1 2UQ
0733 555988
Telephone advice from Disabled Living Advisors. Field workers
nationwide. Issues fact sheets on receipt of SAE.

Birth Centre
37 Coverton Road, London SW17
081 767 8294
Encourages alternatives to 'mechanized' birth.

BLISS (Baby Life Support System)
17–21 Emerald Street, London WC1
071 831 9393
Provides equipment and nurse training for special care baby
units. Also information and support (Blisslink) for parents
whose babies are in special care. Leaflets and information
supplied.

British Agency for Adoption and Fostering (BAAF)
Skyline House, 200 Union Street, London SE1 0LY
071 593 2000
Advice and information to professionals and clients.

British Association for Counselling
1 Regent Place, Rugby CV21 2PJ
0788 550899
Holds directory of suitably qualified counsellors for individuals
or couples.

British Pregnancy Advisory Service (BAPS)
Austy Manor, Wooton Wawen, Solihull, West Midlands B95 6BX
0564 793225
Counselling and treatment for contraception and termination.

Brook Advisory Centres
153a East Street, London SE17 2SD
071 708 1234/1390
Contraceptive advice and counselling for young people.

Caesarian Avoidance Support Scheme
Poplars Farm, Silverleys Green, Halesworth, Suffolk IP19 0QJ
Advice and support for mothers wishing to avoid caesarian delivery.

Catholic Marriage Guidance Council
15 Lansdowne Road, Holland Park, London W11 3AJ
071 727 0141

The Child Bereavement Trust
(Director: Jenni Thomas) Ramworth, Doggett's Wood Lane, Chalfont St Giles, Bucks HP8 4TJ

Compassionate Friends
53 North Street, Bristol BS3 1EN
0272 539639
Support and counselling for bereaved parents.

Cot Death Research and Support
35 Belgrave Square, London SW1X 8QB
071 235 1721/0965

Cruse (Bereavement Care and Support)
Cruse House, 126 Sheen Road, Richmond, Surrey TW9 1UR
081 332 7227 (helpline office hours)
081 940 4818 (administration)
Counselling for all bereaved individuals.

Crysis
BM Crysis, London WC1N 3XX
071 404 5011
Advice and support for parents whose children cry excessively.

Depressives Anonymous
36 Chestnut Avenue, Beverley, North Humberside HU17 9QU
(please send SAE)
0482 860619 (for information)
Support for sufferers and advice for carers.

Depressives Associated
PO Box 1022, London SE1 7QB
081 760 0544 (answerphone)
Information and support for sufferers and their families.

Expectant Mothers Clinic
British School of Osteopathy, 1–4 Suffolk Street, London SW1
071 930 9254
Treatment for postural disorders during pregnancy. Instruction
for partners in massage techniques.

Family Planning Association
27–35 Mortimer Street, London W1N 7RJ
071 636 7866
Advice on all aspects of contraception. Counselling for psychosexual problems.

Family Welfare Association
501–5 Kingsland Road, London E8 4AU
071 254 6251
Independent social work agency for distressed families.

Foresight Charity for Preconceptual Care
28 The Paddock, Godalming, Surrey GU7 1XD
0483 427839
Advice on diet, mineral and vitamin supplementation before
conception. Send SAE for details of local clinics.

Foundation for the Study of Infant Deaths
35 Belgrave Square, London SW1X 8QB
071 235 1721 (24-hour helpline)
071 235 0965 (administration)

Gingerbread
35 Wellington Street, London WC2E 7BN
071 240 0953
Offers help and support to one-parent families. Nationwide self-
help support groups.

Healthrights
Unit 405, Brixton Small Business Centre, 444 Brixton Road,
London SW9 8EJ
071 274 4000 (Ext. 326)
Advises on all aspects of health care, especially maternity.

Homestart Headquarters
2 Salisbury Road, Leicester LE1 7QR
0533 554988
Offers practical help and emotional support to mothers of children aged under five.

Independent Midwives' Association
Nightingale Cottage, Shamblehurst Lane, Botley,
Nr. Southampton SO3 2BY
0703 694429
An association of private midwives who offer a domiciliary service for a fixed fee.

Issue (National Fertility Association Ltd)
509 Aldridge Road, Great Barr, Birmingham B44 8NA
021 344 4414
Self-help organization offering information and support to professionals and clients.

La Leche League
BM 3424, London WC1 6XX
071 242 1278
Breast-feeding advice. Send SAE for information.

LIFE
Life House, Newbold Terrace, Leamington Spa,
Warwickshire CV32 4EA
0926 421587
Practical help for unsupported mothers. Post-abortion counselling.

Maternity Alliance
15 Britannia Street, London WC1 9JP
071 837 1265
Supplies information about healthcare, financial and legal rights. Campaigns for improvements in social support for pregnant women and parents.

Maternity and Health Links
The Old Co-op, 42 Chelsea Road, Easton, Bristol BS5 6AF
0272 558495
Offers support, tuition and interpreting service for non-English speaking mothers.

Maternity Services Liaison Scheme
Brady Centre, 192 Hanbury Street, London E1 5HU
071 377 1064
Support for women of ethnic minorities during pregnancy, labour and postpartum.

Meet-A-Mum Association (MAMA)
58 Malden Avenue, South Norwood, London SE25 4HS
081 656 7318
Self-help groups for mothers feeling socially isolated with young children. Helpful literature.

Miscarriage Association
PO Box 24, Ossett, West Yorkshire WF5 9XG
0924 200799

Multiple Births Foundation
Queen Charlotte's and Chelsea Hospital, Goldhawk Road, London W6 0XG
081 740 3519/3520
Advice, information and support for mothers of multiple births. Advice to professionals.

National Association for Premenstrual Syndrome (NAPS)
PO Box 72, Sevenoaks, Kent TN13 1XQ
0732 741709
Issues information and advice to sufferers.

National Childbirth Trust
Alexandra House, Oldham Terrace, London W3 6NH
081 992 8637
Nationwide organization offering preparation for birth, labour and breast-feeding in small classes. Informative books and pamphlets.

National Council for One-parent Families
255 Kentish Town Road, London NW5
071 267 1361
Advice for single pregnant women and single parents of both sexes.

Newpin
35 Sutherland Square, Walworth, London SE17 3EE
071 703 6326
Support network and drop-in centre for vulnerable families with young children.

NIPPERS (National Information for the Parents of Prematures)
Perinatal Research Unit, St Mary's Hospital, Praed Street, London W2 1NY
071 725 1487

Parentline
Westbury House, 57 Hart Road, Thundersley, Essex SS7 3PD
0268 757077
24-hour answering service for parents under stress. Local groups.

Parents Anonymous
9 Manor Gardens, Islington, London N7
071 263 8918
Confidential telephone support service to parents of problem children.

Parents at Work
77 Holloway Road, London N7 8JZ
071 700 5771
Practical advice on returning to work after childbirth.

PMS Help
PO Box 160, St Albans, Herts AL1 4UQ

Pre-eclamptic Toxaemia Society (PETS)
Ty Iago, High Street, Llanberis, Gwynned, Wales
0286 872477
Support and self-help groups for women with pregnancy-induced hypertension. Newsletter.

RELATE (Marriage Guidance Council)
Herbert Gray College, Little Church Street, Rugby CV21 3AP
0788 573241
Relationship and psychosexual counselling at many local centres.

Samaritans
10 The Grove, Slough, Berks SL1 1QP
0753 532713
24-hour/day support for those in distress. Many local branches: number to be found in local telephone directory.

SANDS (Stillbirth and Neonatal Death Society)
28 Portland Place, London W1N 4DE
071 436 5881
Support and counselling for parents of babies who die at or soon after birth. Telephone contact with other mothers.

Support after Termination for Foetal Abnormality (SATFA)
29/30 Soho Square, London W1V 6JB
071 439 6124
Runs workshops and parents' self-help meetings nationwide. Telephone helpline and newsletter.

Twins and Multiple Births Association (TAMBA)
PO Box 30, Little Sutton, South Wirral L66 1TH
051 348 0020
Parents' support groups.

Women's Health Concern
17 Earls Terrace, London W8 6LP
081 602 6669
Information and advice for those suffering from gynaecological
and obstetric problems. Publications.

Women's Therapy Centre
6 Manor Gardens, London N7 6LA
071 263 6200
Offers individual and group therapy at low cost.

Bibliography

Books Suitable for Health Carers and Women in Pregnancy and Postpartum

Apter T. (1994) *Why women don't have wives: Professional success and motherhood*. Macmillan, London.

Borg S and Lasker J. (1983) *When pregnancy fails*. Routledge and Kegan Paul, London.

Bourne G. (1981) *Pregnancy*. Pan Books, London.

Bradford N. *The well woman's self help directory*. Available from Marie Stopes' Women's Health Clinics.

Bradman T. (1983) *The essential father*. Unwin Hyman, London.

Castro M. (1992) *Homeopathy for mother and baby*. Macmillan, London.

Chalmers B. (1984) *Early parenthood – heaven or hell*. Juta, Cape Town.

Comport M. (1989) *Surviving motherhood: How to cope with postnatal depression*. Ashgrove Press, Bath.

Comport M. (1987) *Towards happy motherhood*. Corgi, London.

Dally A. (1982) *Inventing motherhood – the consequences of an ideal*. Burnett (Hutchinson).

Dix C. (1985) *The new mother syndrome: Coping with postnatal stress and depression*. Allen and Unwin, London.

Dix C. (1989) *Working mothers: You, your career, your child.* Unwin Hyman, London.

Dix C and Sher J. (1985) *Pregnancy: Everything you need to know.* Penguin, Harmondsworth, Middlesex.

Eichenbaum L and Orbach S. (1985) *Understanding women.* Penguin, Harmondsworth, Middlesex.

Friedman R and Gradstein B. (1982) *Surviving pregnancy loss.* Little Brown, Boston MA.

Gieve K. (1989) *Balancing acts – on being a mother.* Virago, London.

Greenberg M. (1985) *The birth of a father.* Continuum, New York.

Greer G. (1984) *Sex and destiny: The politics of human fertility.* Secker and Warburg, London.

Inch S. (1982) *Birthrights: A parents' guide to modern childbirth.* Hutchinson, London.

Katz Rothman B. (1993) *The tentative pregnancy: Prenatal diagnosis and the future of motherhood.* Pandora, London.

Kitzinger S. (1978) *Women as mothers: How they see themselves in different cultures.* Fontana, London.

Kitzinger S. (1991) *Birth over 30.* Sheldon Press, London.

Kitzinger S. (1992) *Breastfeeding your baby.* Dorling Kindersley, London.

Kitzinger S, editor. (1991) *The midwife challenge.* Pandora, London.

Marshall F. (1992) *Coping successfully with your second child.* Sheldon Press, London.

Marshall F. (1993) *Coping with postnatal depression.* Sheldon Press, London.

O'Brien P. (1991) *Your life after birth.* Pandora, London.

Oakley A. (1986) *From here to maternity.* Pelican, Harmondsworth, Middlesex.

Oakley A, McPherson A and Roberts H. (1990) *Miscarriage.* Penguin, Harmondsworth, Middlesex.

Palmer G. (1993) *The politics of breastfeeding.* Pandora, London.

Parke RD. (1981) *Fathering.* Fontana, London.

Parry V. (1993) *The antenatal testing book.* Pan Books Ltd, London.

Phillips A and Rakusen J. (1978) *Our bodies, ourselves.* Penguin, Harmondsworth, Middlesex.

Phillips A, Leap N and Jacobs B. (1991) *Your body, your baby, your life.* Pandora, London.

Price J. (1988) *Motherhood – what it does to your mind.* Pandora, London.

Raphael-Leff J. (1993) *Pregnancy – the inside story.* Sheldon Press, London.

Rich A. (1977) *Of woman born: Motherhood as an experience and institution.* Virago, London.

Rowe D. (1983) *Depression: The way out of your prison.* Routledge and Kegan Paul, London.

Seel R. (1987) *The uncertain father.* Gateway Books, Bath.

Shaevitz M. (1985) *The superwoman syndrome.* Fontana, London.

Shapiro J. (1991) *A child: Your choice.* Pandora, London.

Verney T and Kelly J. (1981) *The secret life of the unborn child.* Sphere, Boston.

Welburn V. (1980) *Postnatal depression.* Fontana, London.

Wesson N. (1987) *Pregnancy and childbirth: Your right to have it your own way.* Thorsons, London.

Books More Suitable for Health Care Professionals

Apfel RJ and Handel MH. (1993) *Madness and loss of motherhood: Sexuality, reproduction and long-term mental illness.* American Psychiatric Press, Washington.

Ball J. (1987) *Reactions to motherhood.* Cambridge University Press, Cambridge.

Brockington IF and Kumar R, editors. (1982) *Motherhood and mental illness.* Academic Press, London.

Cox JL. (1986) *Postnatal depression: A guide for health professionals.* Churchill Livingstone, Edinburgh.

Cox JL, Kumar R, Margison FR, *et al.*, editors. (1986) *Puerperal mental illness*. Duphar Laboratories Ltd, Southampton.

Cox JL, Paykel ES and Page ML, editors. (1989) *Childbirth as a life event*. Duphar Medical Relations, c/o Duphar Laboratories Ltd, Southampton.

Garcia J, Kilpatrick R and Richards M. (1990) *The politics of maternity care – services for childbearing women in the twentieth century*. Clarendon Press, Oxford.

Hall L and Lloyd S. (1989) *Surviving childhood sexual abuse*. The Falmer Press, London and Basingstoke.

Klaus M and Kennell J. (1983) *Bonding*. Mosby, St Louis.

Klompenhouwer J-L. (1992) *Puerperal psychosis*. Horst Publications, Amsterdam.

Kumar R and Brockington IF, editors. (1988) *Motherhood and mental illness 2*. Butterworth, London.

Lewis C. (1986) *Becoming a father*. Open University Press, Milton Keynes.

Lewis C and O'Brien M. (1987) *Reassessing fatherhood*. Sage Publications, London.

Oakley A. (1980) *Women confined: Towards a sociology of childbirth*. Martin Robertson, Blackwell, Oxford.

Raphael-Leff J. (1991) *Psychological processes of childbearing*. Chapman & Hall, London.

Redshaw M, Rivers R and Rosenblatt D. (1985) *Born too soon*. Oxford University Press, Oxford.

Sandler M, editor. (1978) *Mental illness in pregnancy and the puerperium*. Oxford University Press, Oxford.

Tew, S. (1990) *Safer childbirth – a critical history of maternity care*. Chapman & Hall, London.

Video Resources

Postnatal Depression

Corporate Television 1993; 12 minutes.
Designed for use with antenatal classes.
Corporate Television, 44 Ridgeway Avenue, Newport, Gwent NP9 5AH
0633 213280
£50.00 plus VAT.

Postnatal Depression – Who Cares?

Central Television 1984; 28 minutes.
Useful as a teaching aid for midwives and health visitors; also suitable for antenatal and postnatal classes.
Available from Video Resources Unit, Central Television, Broad Street, Birmingham B1 2JP
£25.28. Information booklet also available.

A Question of Depression: The Postnatal Patient

DISTA Psychiatric Education Services 1991; 17 minutes.
More suitable for general practitioners.
Eli Lilly, 0256 485282, or contact local Lilly or DISTA medical representatives.

Newpin – A Lifeline

BBC *Horizon* programme 1989; 50 minutes.
A description of the work of the organization, which offers support to depressed or disadvantaged mothers. Suitable for social workers or those working in primary care. Available to hire.
Newpin, 35 Sutherland Square, Walworth, London SE17 3EE
071 703 6326

Index

Index 243

postnatal depression 93–4
infertility history
  postnatal depression 81, 85
  and pregnancy 10
irritability, postnatal depression
  56–7
isocarboxazid 179

labetalol 185
labour 26–34
  difficulties
    mother-baby relationship
     disorders 142–3, 155
    postnatal depression 83–4,
     85, 96
    puerperal psychosis 117, 128
  father's role 204
  fear of 85
labour room 26–7
Lentizol 177
libido problems, postnatal
  depression 60
Librium 167
LIFE 218
life events, and postnatal
  depression 77, 87, 81
liothyronine 186
lithium 8
  hypothyroidism 186
  puerperal psychosis 116, 124,
   126–7, 128
  side-effects 163, 169–70, 171,
   183–4
lithotomy stirrups 26
lorazepam 181, 182
low mood, postnatal depression
  55–6
L-thyroxine 186
Ludiomil 179

Main, Tom 216
Manerix 179

manic-depressive illness
  medication 170
  and puerperal psychosis 110,
   117, 118
maprotiline hydrochloride 179
Marcé Society 214, 215, 221, 222
marital status
  and postnatal depression 76,
   80
  and puerperal psychosis 117
Marplan 179
masochistic repercussions of
  sexual abuse 149
Maudsley Personality Inventory
  84
medication
  pregnancy 7–8
  psychotropic 186–7
   in breast milk 172–86
   in pregnancy 162–71
  for puerperal psychosis 116,
   123
Meet-a-Mum Association
  (MAMA) 21
Melleril 175
memory problems *see* amnesia
menstruation
  and postnatal depression 79,
   85, 90
  and puerperal psychosis 128
methimazole 186
mianserin 178–9
midazolam 181–2
midwives
  early puerperium 39, 42
  labour 30–1
  postnatal depression 62
  role 212
  sexual abuse survivors 152
  training 214
migraine 41
MIND 218

Printed in the United States
by Baker & Taylor Publisher Services

Printed in the United States
by Baker & Taylor Publisher Services